NOW I UNDERSTAND YOU

NOW I UNDERSTAND YOU

Essays

JOANNA MANNING

Subduction Zone Press

For reprint permissions, contact Subduction Zone Press at info@subductionzonepress.com.

Library of Congress Control Number: 2022904958
ISBN: 978-0-578-39386-5

Cover art provided by Ruth Black, courtesy of Canva.

First Printing, 2022

Contents

Perhaps I know best why it is man alone
who laughs; he alone suffers so deeply
that he had to invent laughter.
—*Friedrich Nietzsche*

Prologue

My father was a hearty laugher. He was given to a kind of wheezy, tearful, riotous outburst when something tickled him, and if you've ever been in the company of someone who has been utterly consumed by a laugh, you know how contagious this is. I have inherited this trait from him, and my family can always sense when I'm about to lose control.

"Here we go," one of them will say as they all break out into anticipatory laughter. Then we let the moment overtake us.

I used to find my father's laughing embarrassing. At the movies, he had a tendency to wait until the audience had quieted after a funny scene, then he'd repeat the punchline and begin his whooping all over again, dragging a few helpless strangers down with him in the process. It is nearly impossible to resist joining in on this kind of unbridled joy. I recognize the beauty of that now.

Some of my fondest memories are of laughing to the point of tears. What prompted the laughing itself has become irrelevant over time. Surrender is what I really savored. A good laugh is second perhaps only to good sex, but if you've been intimate with someone for long enough, you've probably had occasion to do both simultaneously. And it was likely more satisfying than anything else you were trying to do simultaneously, no matter what you were told as a teenager.

As much as I enjoy a tearful laughing fit, at times it will round the corner and morph into actual crying. I am not alone in this, I know. The brain structures responsible for turning laughter into tears are the same ones that prompt us to pinch a cute baby's cheeks or threaten to eat their fat little toes. The brain does not like to be overwhelmed by emotion and will swing the pendulum in the opposite direction to restore a sense of equilibrium. My own emotional pendulum has a wider arc than most, I suppose, but the extreme highs and lows have been a gift in their own way, and instructive: *This, too, shall pass* is as true amid joy as it is in sorrow.

My father struggled mightily to bend that arc toward joy. More than laughing, he loved to make others laugh and was a natural born performer, hitting up open mics and starring in various community theater productions at every opportunity. I seem to have inherited this trait from him as well. When I first tried my hand at stand-up, I finally understood what drew my father to the stage. The high I felt came not from feeling admired when the audience liked my jokes but from feeling that I had *ministered* to people by offering them this escape. It felt almost holy, which was ironic, since most of my act was profane.

The world can feel bleak. For some people, it always feels this way. For my father, the darkness was too deep and all-consuming to escape. This book is my attempt at shining a light into that darkness. And while most of what follows is a light-hearted glimpse into an ordinary life, there is

melancholy here, too. We have to sit in both spaces to appreciate either one. It's a truth stenciled onto wooden signs in
every home décor store across the country: *To enjoy a rainbow,
you have to put up with the rain.* If you have that sign hanging
in your house, however, I have little hope that we could ever
be friends.

I

Make, Model, and Class

Every other Friday, my father picked me up for the weekend in his battered little truck. I don't recall the make or model, just that it was old and white and running on its original spark plugs after well over a hundred thousand miles. The spark plugs' improbable lifespan was one of those peculiar things people tend to brag about when there's not much else in the way of achievements to point out. My father mentioned them several times, often enough for me to remember, perhaps as evidence that at least one thing was working in his favor. That was before his truck caught on fire.

We were driving down Union Avenue in Altoona, Pennsylvania, one afternoon—the same as we had every other Friday in the past—when smoke began billowing up around us and snaking its way into the windows. I was about ten years old and hardly an expert in auto mechanics, but even I could tell that something was amiss.

People began honking to alert us to the obvious fact that we were driving blind through our own personal smoke cloud. A jogger ran up alongside us and yelled through the open window, "Hey, Buddy! Your truck's on fire!"

My father nodded and waved, the picture of calm. The next thing I remember, he was telling me to jump out. His voice was so measured I could hardly believe he meant it.

"Are you serious?" I asked.

"Jump out," he said again, this time with more urgency. He stretched out across the cabin, opened the door, and pushed me out before making a turn onto a side street and crashing into the back of a van. Then, as if from nowhere, a throng of people arrived on the scene, surrounding the truck and dousing the flames with their garden hoses.

I was dazed but unharmed. As I stumbled around the crash site, I spotted my friend Jennifer Donnelley from across the crowd, but she was too busy selling candy bars from a school fundraiser to the onlookers to notice me. I have to admire her for her opportunism now, but at the time I was more than a little bit irked that she was stealing all of the business. My own candy was in the smoldering truck, and I figured I should have been able to reap some of the profits considering I was the child just thrust from that steaming pile of metal everyone had gathered to gawk at. Now they were all standing around wiping chocolate from their open mouths, and I was not a penny richer.

When the initial shock of the accident wore off, I remember feeling completely exhilarated by the experience. I had just jumped from a moving vehicle without so much as a single lesson in Hollywood stunt performance and somehow had miraculously survived. No one had to know that we had already slowed to about five miles per hour when I was pushed out or that the truck wasn't exactly engulfed in flames. For all I knew, we were just on the verge of a gas tank explosion. I spent so much time as a kid preoccupied with the mere prospect of dying that to have even the slightest brush with death gave me a high I'd only previously felt from my codeine-laced cough syrup.

I'm not sure how many times I uttered the words "I jumped out of a burning truck" in the ensuing weeks, but I'm sure I wore the phrase thin. Had I grown up in anywhere other than a working-class town, the story might have outed my family as a *certain kind* of people—namely, the kind who could only afford to drive shitty trucks that would spontaneously combust on occasion. It's a common enough tale among my brethren.

The ubiquitous break-down story had the same subtext as my stories of eating mayonnaise sandwiches or getting paid a quarter to fetch my grandfather cans of PBR during his Friday-night card games, or any anecdote that mentioned drug abuse and alcoholism or the double-wide trailer I spent my formative years in, even if that double-wide was only intended to be a placeholder for the farm house that never came to be. Then again, the house-that-never-got-built story is in the same vein as the others—the poverty porn of rural decline, everything people of means and urban elites ever need to know to form an opinion about the working and lower classes.

Not that many of these elites existed in the railroad town where I lived—Altoona was a bit of a cultural vacuum. Most of us were in the same socio-economic sphere, so there weren't many people who would have cared much about our status in the first place. That also meant the van my father crashed into was likely in a similar state of disrepair as his flaming truck. There was no self-consciousness about the accident in its aftermath, merely commiseration.

"What can you do?" I can hear the van owner saying with a knowing shrug. "Sometimes your brake line just catches fire."

Nevertheless, I would have been wise to have kept my mouth shut about any of my childhood experiences later in life. But as a certain class of person, I had never learned this kind of restraint at home, and Roosevelt Junior High was hardly a finishing school for the socially ambitious. We were, after all, the Rough Riders for God's sake.

Poor kids rarely realize they're poor. It's not until they become adults that they come to view their childhood through the lens of class. At least that was the case for me. My basic needs had always been met, and I'd come to understand that to want much more would be a kind of sin, so I was perfectly content to not want anything. I still don't derive much joy from material things, and I consider that an unintended blessing of a lean childhood.

It also helped that I grew up in a small town, which was actually more egalitarian than the big city solely because there weren't many private schools separating the haves from the have-nots from an early age. There were plenty of Catholic schools around, but they didn't cater to the children from monied families necessarily, they mostly just weeded out the Italians.

The professional people largely sent their children to the local public schools, and we mixed according to our abilities. If you happened to be a poor kid who was intelligent in a way that was measurable on a standardized test, you could mingle with the upper crust with ease. It was our own fantasy meritocracy.

I went to college, on an ROTC scholarship, sincerely believing this meritocracy was an absolute truth and held the key to social and intellectual mobility. As long as I could drop Derrida or Lacan into conversation or quote Cicero in his native Latin, I knew I would always have a home with the cultural elite. But there was also this unrefined side of me—the we-who-dump-old-appliances-into-ravines side—that helped me survive my years in the military but threatened to out me to the intellectuals I so longed to belong with. I spent most of my twenties trying to square these parts of myself.

Though academic types tended to overlook my rough edges as long as my ideas were interesting enough, I found other circles to be somewhat less forgiving. The first time I recall feeling a real sense of class consciousness was after I joined the Junior League, at the tail end of an acceptable age to do so. I was peripherally aware of the League's reputation as a place for well-heeled women to gather together to help the less fortunate, but I joined a chapter in the über-casual Pacific Northwest, a place where I assumed the class aspects of the League would be shunned in favor of its mission of female empowerment. This was not entirely the case.

The majority of the women came from affluent backgrounds and possessed a refinement I admired but didn't feel intimidated by, perhaps because I, myself, was too unrefined to know that I should have felt intimidated. Their world had not been my world growing up, but I assumed I had earned my golden ticket into their social circle by way of an advanced degree and extensive world travel. They were bound to find me charming.

I was amused by the thought that I was possibly the only woman in history to have ever simultaneously belonged to the Junior League and a bowling league, and I fancied myself part of a one-woman revolution, intent on turning class on its head by straddling these worlds and proving I could belong in both.

Over time, however, I began to notice the League women and their ilk would tell me that they'd find my "candor" refreshing, that they could always count on me to be "real." Though they'd claim to appreciate the "vulnerability" I brought to the table by way of a lack of filter, I eventually realized these were subtle ways of mocking me, even if they *did* appreciate, on some level, that I would always speak my mind. It helped that I was speaking with an intelligent coarseness, but I was coarse nonetheless.

As the old saying goes, you can toss the girl out of a burning truck, but you can't take a burning truck out of the girl. Any illusions I'd been sustaining about social mobility turned out to be just that—illusions. People who are born into their money can sniff out social climbers in an instant, as if they can still smell the Spam on our breath. No amount of education or travel can compensate for that. And frankly, I no longer care. I'd rather be candid and real and vulnerable and myself. I'm far more entertaining that way.

But getting to that place of acceptance was a long road. When I first understood that my openness with the Junior League set was not the subject of delight but of derision, I felt humiliated. How long had I been embarrassing myself while people humored me? I came home from a meeting one night in tears, telling my husband I felt like some kind of exotic zoo animal the women only kept around for their entertainment. We sat in silence for a few minutes as he eyed me with sympathy.

"Is it because you're wearing stripes?" he finally asked.

In that moment, I could at least feel heartened that I had married well.

2

Screen Times

The problem with being married to a man who grew up without television is that every time you stick your face into a metal sieve and begin reciting the "magic mirror" portion of *Romper Room*, he'll just stare at you as if he's assessing you for signs of a stroke.

"Romper stomper bomper boo!" I said, creeping into the room where my husband and son were watching football. *Romper Room* was such a staple of my youth that I still can't pass up the opportunity to do the magic mirror routine any time I have my hands on something circular. My performance with the sieve was met with blank stares, however, so I had to pull up an old clip of the show on my phone just to prove I hadn't been day drinking.

"*This* is what you watched every day?" my son asked, his face scrunched.

I nodded. "I always hoped she'd see me in the magic mirror and say my name," I told him. "She never did though."

My husband touched my arm. "That's the saddest thing I've ever heard."

I could only shrug my shoulders. I didn't need his pity. *He* was the one with the gaping television-shaped hole in his heart that I could never hope to fill, no matter how tirelessly I worked to recreate the programming from our youth. So, I returned to the kitchen with my sieve, happily reciting the rest of the *Romper Room* lines to myself: *Tell me, tell me, tell me, do.*

I should clarify that my husband's parents *owned* a television when he was a kid. They weren't philosophically opposed to it or fearful of its corrupting influence on the youth. It was a simple problem of geography that kept them from actually watching much TV.

Chad grew up in a small Colorado mountain town that was nestled into the base of Pike's Peak at a dizzying elevation of 8,000 feet. The town didn't have paved roads let alone cable, so no one could tune into much more than the three main networks unless they were willing to shell out a hefty sum for a satellite dish large enough to communicate with alien life while beaming *60 Minutes* into their living rooms.

To hear my husband talk of his childhood though, you'd think he'd been too busy traipsing off into the woods with his rifle like a mini Davy Crockett to have bothered with something as dull as television in the first place. It just wasn't important to him. Besides, it probably would have been difficult to enjoy watching *Bugs Bunny* after spending an afternoon skinning rabbits.

I, on the other hand, can hardly imagine a scene from my childhood that did not have a television in it. It was always on in the background, even if no one was watching, probably as a way to keep my mother company while my father was away during the week. And for me—an only child growing up alone in the country—the characters on screen often served as my only companions. I had to form relationships one way or another, even fictitious ones.

Television was one part friend, one part babysitter, and I loved spending time with it even more than I enjoyed spending time with its real-life human equivalents. I watched game shows in the mornings and re-runs of 1970s sitcoms every afternoon without fail, which were both educational in their own way. *The Price is Right* taught me about economics, and the *Laverne and Shirley* theme song taught me my first Yiddish words. I was perhaps the only five-year-old in town who could effectively kvetch about the price of groceries whenever I'd accompany my mother to the store.

Mork and Mindy was one of my favorite shows in the afternoon lineup. I had always been confused by Mork's "until next week" sign-off until my mother explained that the original show only aired once a week. I took the news as one might hear word that a loved one had been shipped off to war. It was an unthinkable horror to me. *How could I ever wait an entire week to see my favorite show*, I wondered? I might have had a mild addiction.

Maybe mild is understated. When I was young, barely a toddler by my mother's account, I used to get up in the middle of the night and insist on watching TV. The fact that the stations stopped broadcasting at around midnight didn't deter me. I would tromp down the stairs, park myself in front of our floor model Zenith and stare at the test pattern on the screen for a half hour or so, all while my parents looked on, never once thinking of calling a child psychologist.

The television had a hypnotic appeal. It still does. Once screens became palm-sized and widely available, their addictive quality became readily apparent. But that's an altogether different issue. Though I clearly spent a bit too much time absorbed in these fictitious worlds on the screen, I also escaped into books and imaginative play and outdoor adventures around the farm. Television soothed me, nothing more. It was familiar and predictable in a way that life couldn't always be counted on to be. And when I finally learned more productive ways to soothe myself, that's what I did.

Still, the hold it had on me ran deep. The first time I watched *Sesame Street* with my first child, the theme song stirred up such an intense feeling of nostalgia that I began sobbing, as if I'd finally been reconnected with that loved one who'd shipped off years before. I tried to examine my reaction, but the emotions were complex. Was I yearning for the innocence of childhood, for those carefree, idle days? Had I been attacked by a dog while watching the show as a child? It was impossible to say. I finally just chalked the crying fit up to hormones and settled in for a visit with my old friends on the street.

These days, it's nearly impossible to escape being passively entertained by a screen. There's almost no choice in the matter. There are televisions at the gas pump and at each exam chair at the dentist's office. I've even seen them at some grocery store checkout lanes. As a child, I would have been overjoyed by this. Now that I'm older and more content to examine my interior life when I find myself standing still in the world, the constant chatter annoys me.

Were it not for the screens, we might use these moments to talk to the people who are standing around us in real life. Maybe it would be wise not to lead with that old *Romper Room* question—*Are you having a special day today, friend?*—but it wouldn't hurt to turn away from the technology and toward each other, to reach out and learn a stranger's name every now and then. You never know how long a person has been waiting to really be seen, even without a magic mirror.

3

Save Me

When the Faith Non-Denominational Church of Hyndman, Pennsylvania, handed out salvation, I did not attend. If I could pinpoint a single event that served as a catalyst for my lifelong anxiety problems, it might very well be this one: I missed church on the day the Sunday school teachers had chosen to lead the children through the Sinner's Prayer, which was a simple little ritual that committed their young lives to God and spared them from burning in the eternal fires of Hell.

When I showed up to Sunday school a few weeks later and heard rumblings of this salvation business, I asked the teacher if I could be saved as well. This should have been simple enough to accomplish, but she outright refused, citing some policy that she could only save the children once a year. Maybe this was a draconian way to encourage church attendance—and to be fair, my parents were fond of sleeping in—but it hardly seemed the Christian thing to do.

I knew precious little about God at this point in my life, but

I was familiar enough with the fire-and-brimstone message of the Old Testament and had seen artists' renditions of Hell in my mother's family Bible. As I stood there in that church basement thinking about what it meant to be "unsaved," I thought of my mother's Bible illustrations and of those poor sinners' souls being tossed into the lake of fire. Suddenly, I felt a bit skeptical of the lyrics to "Jesus Loves Me." Jesus may, but his father was a wild card. I was in a pickle.

I had no choice but to place my faith in my classmates. I walked around the room, badgering them for more information on how to be saved, hoping it was something that I could do on my own. This turned out to be a shrewd move. When I asked a neighbor boy what I needed to do, he simply told me. He gave up the keys to the kingdom without even putting up a fight or offering some snide commentary about my church attendance record.

"Just say that you love Jesus and stuff," he said.

That was it? I could hardly believe it was so simple. Apart from the "and stuff" part, which I took to be verbal filler on the part of my friend, not an indication that Jesus wanted me to be a capitalist, I felt sure I could prove my devotion. I didn't take time to reflect on what this meant or why I should love this man. I didn't ask if there were any strings attached or first-born children to sign away. I was young. I did it because I was told to, in much the same way I would dutifully hug elderly relatives whose embraces left me choking on Chantilly powder and Old Spice.

Armed with this new knowledge, I committed myself to earning my salvation. I sang little ditties about loving Jesus. I recited his name like a mantra. I scribbled "I-heart-Jesus" on all of the paper I could find. After a few weeks, confident that I had dispensed with my obligations, my fear of damnation began to fade.

But old fears are quick to be revived.

The timeline is a bit fuzzy now, but sometime after my initial complications with getting into heaven through active faith, I was introduced to the concept of passive salvation through baptism. My parents had failed to baptize me when I was born, leaving me in a precarious state of spiritual limbo. Since I had already taken the side door to being saved, I figured I couldn't risk missing out on this, too. So when my mother had planned to be baptized by immersion in a nearby river, I begged her to ask the preacher to include me.

He sat across from us in our living room, sipping iced tea while he considered the request. My mother talked. He sipped. She talked some more. He nodded. Finally, he told my mother I was too young to know what I was entering into. My heart sank.

The world had conspired to send me to Hell.

From that moment on, I was obsessed with dying, a fear that gave birth to a few peculiar rituals. I still remember believing that my index fingers were always pointing in the direction I would go when I died. No matter how good or faithful I had been while here, dying with those fingers pointed toward the ground was a guaranteed high-speed train ticket to Hell. With this in mind, I made a habit of clasping my hands together in front of my face, pointing my forefingers to the heavens. People would occasionally ask what I was doing, but even back then I was at least partially aware of the absurdity of this practice, so I never gave an answer.

If there were pediatric mental institutions back then, I probably belonged in one. Some of these behaviors were borderline psychotic. For a while I was convinced that my saliva was poisoned and took to spitting it out whenever my mother wasn't looking. Poisoned saliva was the perfect crime, a murder plot of such genius only God could devise it. I was convinced that the Almighty would try to take me precisely while my soul was still in jeopardy, and looking back now, this fear was not completely unfounded. There was a lot of smiting going on in the Old Testament, and God was not always especially kind to children.

Religion brought me no peace as a child, only mortal terror. I had been cut off from God and consigned to the Devil, and it all felt weirdly personal. The Sinner's Prayer is all of five lines that take no more than 30 seconds to recite, but my Sunday school teacher seemed put out by the very suggestion that she say the words with me. You'd have thought I was her deadbeat husband demanding a beer from the fridge instead of a little kid living in fear for her immortal soul.

To make matters worse, I had to witness my mother's baptism, even though I had been excluded from this ritual myself. I remember standing on the riverbank, cloaked in the filth of my unsaved soul, screaming as I watched the preacher push my mother under the water. I had become suspicious of everyone by that time, and the whole affair looked more like murder than salvation to me.

As an adult, I understand that the church didn't *set out* to scar me for life, nor did it treat me with deliberate malice; it was just unusually prescriptive regarding matters of eternity. I was not the only one to suffer because of this kind of legalism. Years later, my dying grandmother would be denied baptism by a hospital chaplain who claimed it wasn't necessary, that God knew what was in her heart. She said nothing, but her eyes mirrored my own old fears. What harm could have come from a few words, a sprinkle of water, earthly things to soothe the mortal mind?

But ceremony is fraught, too. I can draw a straight line from religious ritual to the compulsive rituals I developed as a young child—ones that persisted into adulthood—to pacify my anxieties about dying. If religious rituals could secure eternal salvation, I reasoned, then secular ones could somehow manage to stave off death in the first place. The thought process didn't have to make sense. It just had to make my palms stop sweating.

Despite these early difficulties with my parents' church, I didn't give up on religion right away. If God truly was the father of my soul, then his seeming indifference was bound to condemn me to a life with the worst kind of daddy issues. This was a relationship I felt I had to repair, even if, by all indications, it appeared that God was just not that into me. So I kept on trying. And I kept on seeking. I am a seeker to this day. I even answer the door when the Mormons come calling.

~

The other day, I was driving my kids home from school when we passed by a church that had put "Where have you found God today?" on its reader board. It was a quiet moment in the car, each of us lost in our own individual thoughts, so I began to consider the question. Where had I felt attuned to something greater than myself that day? Where had I been able to feel the interconnectedness of this life? In the car, with my children. In the calm waters of the Puget Sound. In conversation with a friend. I could name any number of things. Just then, my daughter broke the silence.

"You know that sign outside of the church," she said, "the one that asks where you've found God today?"

I was pleased to think that she had been performing this mental exercise as well. But there was a hint of mischief in her voice, so I was eager to hear what she had been thinking.

"Yes, I was just thinking about it actually," I said. "Were you?"

"I pictured an old man with a white beard hiding behind a tree," she said.

My son snorted. "Like he was playing hide-and-seek?" They both began to giggle before my daughter continued.

"Then he jumped out from behind it and said, 'Hey, how could you not see me over here?'"

It was such a ridiculous thought, that this bearded robed man would spend his days jump scaring us from the trees, that we couldn't help but laugh.

Maybe there was something to what my daughter was envisioning. Maybe God is all around, hiding in plain sight. Maybe I'd never been looking in the right places. But in the car that day, I finally understood how God is always with us, and that in our laughter was a spark of the divine.

4

Unlocking Your Unlimited Potential

While ordinary pre-teen girls in the 1980s spent their weekends at the mall buying stacks of cheap bangles and hot-pink feather earrings from Claire's, I was in Waldenbooks spending my birthday money on guided meditation tapes. I'm not sure how I even discovered the world of audio relaxation and subliminal messaging. I was a high-strung kid for sure, but I wasn't trying to kick a pack-a-day smoking habit at age 11. The tapes were advertised as "self-hypnosis," which I can only imagine held some kind of mystical appeal to me at the time. But if I was disappointed to discover I wasn't going to be hypnotized into a better, more popular version of myself, I can't recall. All I know is that once I had Barrie Konicov's soothing voice in my ear, gently coaching me in the practice of power breathing, I soon found I couldn't go to sleep without him.

Konicov was an interesting character. A marketing man by

training, he began doing hypno-therapy for weight loss and smoking cessation in the 1970s, and he recorded his sessions so that his patients could practice their self-hypnosis skills at home. When those tapes proved to be popular, he formed Potentials Unlimited, offering a broad menu of tapes for people who were looking to improve their self-confidence or hone their psychic abilities. Bolstered by the growing popularity of the self-help industry, Konicov soon became a millionaire who used his wealth to fund a run for political office on the Libertarian ticket. Though he failed in his political ambitions, he developed something of a cult following for his anti-tax views, solidifying his status as folk hero when he was arrested for his refusal to file federal income taxes all through the mid-90s.

None of these unsavory bits had yet come to pass when Konicov was talking me to sleep each night, though his tapes had already ventured into New Age territory that should have served as a warning about his general character. One of his more popular recordings offered to help people recover memories of their past lives so that they could heal the trauma they carried over into this life. How he professed to do this with only a three-week credential from the Ethical Hypnosis Training Center of New Jersey is anyone's guess. But I can't blame him for diving into reincarnation, given the popularity Shirley MacLaine had brought to the subject with her memoir *Out on a Limb*, even if it did undermine his credibility a touch. He was simply tapping into the ethos of the time. And remember—he was a salesman, not a shaman.

Once I'd worn out my guided meditation tape, I turned my attention not to one of the practical subjects like building self-confidence or conversational skills, things that could have helped me actually make friends at school—no, I decided I wanted to learn how to astral project.

If you had a normal childhood that didn't involve being hypnotized by a New Age cult leader as you drifted off to sleep each night, allow me to explain astral projection to you. Some people believe it is possible to deliberately induce an out-of-body experience, consciously separating the soul, or "astral body," from its human prison so that it might go on all kinds of delightful spiritual misadventures through space-time, all the while remaining tethered to the physical body by an infinitely flexible silver cord. Maybe I used to do this regularly in a past life. Maybe it was the subliminal messaging in my first tape that led me to such an esoteric subject. Whatever the reason, I fell victim to my first huckster, happily forking over my own money for the chance to let my soul run wild while I slept.

My desire to escape my own body was probably a typical feeling of pre-adolescence, though how this desire manifested was admittedly strange. But I often felt desperate to be set apart from a world that didn't seem to embrace me. I had an extraordinarily lonely life as a young child, my formative years spent on a small farm with only the animals and my imaginary friends as playmates. Later, when my mother and I had moved to town after my parents divorced, I spent my weekends being shuttled back and forth between my parents' homes rather than spending them at sleepovers or playdates, so I never had much opportunity to learn how to relate to people, and I never had anyone to point out just how strange some of my interests actually were. I only had this older man's voice in my ear each night, assuring me that all things were possible with concentrated effort and belief.

If I wanted to have friends in school, you never would have known it. I did myself no favors by putting my eccentricities on display for my classmates to see and ridicule, without so much as a hint of self-consciousness about it. While other kids gave presentations on ballet and art and Lego engineering for the "how-to" speeches we were assigned in the seventh grade, I had selected astral projection as my topic. I was quick to note at the outset of my speech that I had not yet achieved this feat myself, but I confidently outlined the steps I had learned from Mr. Konicov during our nightly sessions, and I answered my classmates' questions with an air of authority that came from being the only one of my kind in the room.

My English teacher—God bless her—she knew me to be a good kid from my work on the school newspaper, so she was polite enough about the speech itself, but I'm sure I was the talk of the teachers' lounge for a few days after that performance.

Toward the end of high school, when I had finally set aside my more unusual pastimes in the interest of making friends, I was recounting the astral projection story at a party, cringing all the while, when a flash of recognition suddenly overcame my best friend's face.

"Oh my God! You were that weird girl!" he said.

"*Were?*" I said, raising an eyebrow at him as if to say *What's changed?* Then we all broke down laughing, swapping stories of our own individual embarrassments, which of course were legion, painful as adolescence can be. For the first time in my life, sitting around laughing with my friends about our quirks, I felt understood. They had seen me, recognized my weirdness—maybe even commiserated with it—and loved me just the same. It was liberating.

I hadn't thought about any of this in years until I happened upon an article that touted a 4-4-8 breathing technique as a cure-all for stress. I immediately recognized the exercise from the guided meditation tapes of my childhood—breathe in for four counts, hold for four counts, then slowly exhale, mentally counting backwards from eight—and I suddenly had to see if these tapes were still available online. It only took a few minutes for me to find the Potentials Unlimited website, complete with a few audio samples of the tapes I once played nightly.

As soon as I heard Konicov's voice say *Hello. Greetings and welcome,* I was a child again, nestled into the canopy bed at my father's house, my pink Sony Walkman at my side. I may never have learned the art of astral projection, but I learned how to time travel in that moment, all of the intervening decades gone, the stress of time and the world draining from my body the moment my old friend said the word *relax.* He had been a genuine therapist for me in his own way, helping me find the calm center to a world that often seemed filled with danger and turmoil. It's unfortunate that he faced a certain amount of disgrace in his later years, but I suppose it's possible to be both villain and hero in our own stories: villain to the IRS, saving grace for a lonely kid. It just goes to show that no one is one-dimensional, especially within the astral plane. Of all the things Mr. Konicov taught me, I know that much to be true.

5

All Signs Point to Death

My dog has taken to sniffing my armpit in such an intense way that I have come to believe he is busy detecting cancer or some other serious disease through the chemicals in my sweat. Never mind that I have watched this dog run head-long into a fence post at full speed while chasing a biker, I've somehow convinced myself he's gifted enough to save lives with his nose. I don't even know if cancer sniffing dogs are real or if the story was just some junk science that had made the news a few years back, but the logic doesn't matter to my brain in either case. Once the anxiety has been triggered, logical thought processes cease. Then the reptile brain has a field day.

If you've ever wondered what living with anxiety looks like, consider this scene: I'm lying in bed trying to read when my dog sticks his nose in my armpit, sniffing aggressively, and instead of wondering if I should shower, I immediately think, *Well of course I have cancer and isn't it a shame that I won't see the children grow up and will Chad be able to find a nice woman who will love them and keep my picture on the mantle and what will poor* Rosie *do, my sensitive little child who already worries about things like nothingness and eternity, what will my long decline and painful death do to her?* And before I know it, I'm tearing up a little, and my heart is racing, and my palms are sweating so much that my dog's fur sticks to my hand in a damp mat as I pet him.

It's the feel of wet dog hair in my hand that finally lifts me to the surface of this particular avalanche, and I can begin to engage the logical part of my brain again and calm myself. These kinds of racing thoughts are a hallmark of obsessive-compulsive disorder, a fun little mental quirk I have lived with for as long as I can remember.

Though I'm sure there's a genetic component to my problem, environment almost certainly had a role in fomenting my obsession with death and dying. My first church preached almost exclusively about the afterlife and made it clear that I had a better-than-average chance of suffering for eternity once I drifted off into my final sleep. But apart from the fear mongering this church traded in, I had personal brushes with death that I was too young to fully understand, and the closest thing to counseling a kid had access to at the time was the ABC *Afterschool Special*. So, I was left to process these deaths alone: Within a short time of each other, my uncle, at only 21 years old, ended his life with a shotgun, and my cousin, my same age and a playmate from my earliest memories, died of cancer. I don't know that I ever experienced that blissful period of childhood when death is either a completely foreign concept or something exclusively reserved for the elderly. It was a very real and present force in my life, always lurking in the shadows, ready to claim whoever happened to pass by. The arbitrary nature of it all still nags at me.

This obsession with death was all-consuming. Even sleep couldn't keep it at bay. In one of the very first dreams I can recall, I was a corpse myself, some figure from history we'd been learning about in school, someone long dead and reduced to bones in the dirt. I can remember every detail about the room I was in when I woke up from that little horror film —the way the moonlight filtered through the window of my parents' room, which constellations were visible in the night sky—everything.

Over time, I developed ways to quiet my mind when these thoughts would get to be too intrusive. My methods were, clinically speaking, compulsions. I'd find a word on a sign or in a book and rearrange the letters into a specific number of other words, in doing so securing some kind of cosmic protection for myself. I'd do something similar with numbers, manipulating them until they became "good" numbers, which, for reasons I could never articulate, were always odd—usually 3, 9, or 11.

Other behaviors slipped into compulsions over time. Every day after school for almost the entirety of my high-school career, for example, I would sit down with the morning paper, turn to the obituary page, and average the age of death for the day. What likely began as an idle diversion soon became a solemn obligation. I had begun to believe that if I failed to do these calculations each afternoon, I risked landing myself on the obituary page as well, so I continued faithfully in my self-appointed work. The stakes were too high not to.

With all of these compulsions, I couldn't do anything else

until I had finished the task I had prescribed for myself because—and this may be the part that "normal" people might not be able to fully understand—*some misfortune awaited me if I didn't perform these tasks.*

Of course, that *some misfortune* in the form of death always awaits me. It awaits everyone. There's no escaping death, and no ritual will ever protect me from it. That's the logical brain, fully engaged. That's the brain that reflects on the words of Seneca, who wrote in his *Moral Letters*, "It is ruinous for the soul to be anxious about the future and miserable in advance of misery. . ." That's the brain I've put on a Crossfit regimen of cognitive behavioral therapy for years and years. That's also the brain that enjoys a cheat day every now and then, thus the belief in a cancer sniffing dog.

Fortunately, this disorder of mine has taken on a softer tone through the years. Though I've managed to shed most of the compulsions of my youth, I still find myself performing a few relatively innocuous rituals to calm myself from time to time. I recite the same few lines of poetry during takeoff every time I fly in order to keep the plane aloft, for example (a vital service that has yet to be acknowledged by my pilot husband). And before having children, I'd still try to impose order on my life by arranging my physical space *just so,* but I've managed to temper that in order to retain my overall sanity. I no longer find I have to perform these rituals every day as a matter of routine. The tentative peace I've made with the inevitability of dying has made this possible.

Still, every so often something will trigger an attack of obsessive thinking that will get the better of me. It's most often my husband, who has thus far lived his life seemingly unaware of his own mortality. As we sat down to breakfast one morning, on the eve of a surgery I had been dreading, he decided to relay a few medical horror stories that he had heard from one of his co-workers the night before. There was the tale of a man who had nearly died of sepsis after a fairly routine procedure and another of a woman who had died of necrotizing fasciitis after she had scraped herself up in a fall from her mountain bike. I put down my coffee and just stared at him.

"Hi. I'm Joanna," I said. "I don't believe we've met."

After nearly two decades together, I thought he might have figured out that nothing good could come from giving me this sort of information. I didn't need a fresh reminder of the capriciousness of life. I had already convinced myself that the anesthesiologist was accidentally going to kill me before my surgery even began, but this breakfast conversation forced me to consider that even if I woke up from the procedure, some kind of insidious infection would be waiting to finish the job. I couldn't seem to put that thought aside, and before long, a familiar and persistent feeling of doom settled over me as we ate.

The feeling became so persistent over the next few hours that I took a few measures to shield myself from any post-humous shame, beginning with the most obvious potential source of embarrassment—my internet search history. I generally don't search for anything too salacious, but I imagine my search terms might at times be confounding. Why, one might wonder while perusing my history after my death, was I searching "duck penis" and "federal deficit tracker" in the same day, let alone within minutes of each other? I had my reasons, naturally, reasons I'd be happy to explain if I were not dead. But in this worst-case-scenario I wouldn't be around to defend myself, and the living would certainly take liberties with this information. It just seemed prudent to delete everything in advance.

There's something about making specific preparations for death that I have always found to be oddly calming, which is, I imagine, a compulsion in itself. I had high-risk pregnancies, and before my daughter was born, I wrote out detailed instructions for my husband about how and where to scatter my ashes after I inevitably died in childbirth. There were specific places that were meaningful to me that I wanted the children to experience, and I described, at length, what was special about each place. It comforted me to think they would have this way to know me in some small way if they lost me in their early childhood.

Chad laughed when I told him what I was doing, not because he was trying to be insensitive, or because my plan was the general plot to the movie *Elizabethtown*, but because these kinds of thoughts just never occur to him.

"It would be really interesting to see our brains side-by-side in an MRI," I said in a huff. "You know, to see the differences in how men and women respond to anxiety triggers." Chad didn't find this idea even remotely compelling.

"I think you'd be disappointed to see how little of the male brain lights up," he said.

He's probably right. I don't know if this is the difference between us specifically or between men and women in general, but it seems to me that men hold fast to their youthful feelings of invincibility far longer than women do and likely worry less as a result. They also die sooner because of this trait, so I'm not so sure I should be envious.

I'm still trying to strike a balance between these two extremes of indifference and obsession. Exercise has become a useful substitute for compulsive rituals, as has meditation. The Stoics have been good friends to me as well. They tend to be described nowadays as the "original cognitive behavioral therapists," and that's not too far from the truth. I'm making better progress with them than I have with some counselors I've had through the years, but I've always deferred to the authority of older men, even long dead ones.

I no longer obsess about death the way I did when I was younger. Age has brought with it a certain amount of resignation, and with that, peace. That said, I tend to sleep better every time I clear my internet search history.

6

A Valentine for My ENT

In retrospect, I might have been a bit too earnest in how I professed my love for my doctor, but we'll get to that. I had recently had surgery on my septum, and I was back in the doctor's office the day before my scheduled follow-up appointment, begging to have the splints removed from inside my nose. The recovery hadn't been painful necessarily, merely uncomfortable, but while pain can be managed, discomfort must simply be endured. Endurance was never my strong suit.

The splints made it difficult to breathe, eat, and sleep, and they caused a fair amount of postnasal drip that I was certain was actually cerebral spinal fluid leaking from my brain. In general, I felt sick with a terrible head cold, though I wasn't sick at all, and I was desperate to feel well again.

The doctor agreed to remove the splints early. He numbed the inside of my nose, stuck a pair of forceps into a nostril, and told me to breathe out with some force. I had assumed the splints were about the size of a thimble, so I hadn't been worried about having them removed, but the way the doctor

braced his free hand against my shoulder should have prepared me for what he was about to yank from my body.

What emerged from my face were two silicone tubes, each
roughly the size of my index finger, which were both set atop
a large oval of more silicone. There had been so much pressure
in my nasal cavity that the sensation of my face emptying was
not unlike the feeling of giving birth (which I recall, for some
reason, as the feeling of a wet seal slipping from my body).

I was so overwhelmed with relief and possibly a touch
manic from the sudden rush of oxygen to my brain that I
blurted out "I love you," looking the good doctor right in the
eye, which, I'll concede, might have been a bit intense. His
face flushed, and he shifted his gaze to the floor, so I tried to
backtrack a bit and make a joke about the platonic nature of
my feelings.

There I was in the exam chair, giddy and on the verge of
fainting from the sight of my bloody nasal splints, awkwardly
crooning *I love youuuuuu, platonically love youuuuuu* to the
tune of Olivia Newton John's song "I Honestly Love You."
Just a week before, this man had witnessed me crying quietly
on the operating table and advising anyone within earshot to
check my vitals, since I was having a panic attack that I was
certain was going to interfere with my body's response to an-
esthesia. Now, without the handy excuse of being under the
influence of narcotics, I was singing him a platonic love song.
Overall, I had not been making the best impression.

But for the rest of the day, I was in love with the world,
and the world was in love with me. After the appointment,
I wandered around my neighborhood, savoring the unseason-
ably warm and sunny November day. It felt like walking

through a movie scene. I could practically hear music in the air as I made my way down the street, greeting everyone cheerily as I passed. I flashed a double-finger point at the mailman. "Hey there, Steve! Great day to be alive, amiright?" I might have high-fived a few strangers, kissed a few babies. I was ecstatic to the point of being high. Such was the effect my ENT had on me.

As it tends to happen with love, however, that initial high faded, and I'm now content to let the doctor prod me every six months or so. Life carries on. Still, every time I take a deep, unobstructed breath of the crisp winter air, I recall that intoxicating rush of my first full breaths after surgery, and I know that at least for that one day, the love I felt was real.

7

A Modern Proposal

Ricky Martin was my first boyfriend. We got together every Saturday morning, sometime between *The Smurfs* and *Schoolhouse Rock*. He had perfectly feathered hair and plaintive brown eyes and fabulous satin jumpsuits that I coveted for myself. I liked that he resembled the gymnast Mary Lou Retton, because I also admired her *and* her patriotic leotards. God bless America. I loved Ricky so much I didn't even mind that he was in a Latin boy band that translated to "beef stomach" in English. When we danced and sang together, the rest of the world fell away. Saturdays with my wholesome Spanish boyfriend were some of the best days of my young life. But like so many girls before me, I was eventually lured away by a bad boy. His name was George Michael.

When George sang about faith and freedom, I knew my conservative Christian parents would be able to look past the earring and the leather to see him for the good man I knew him to be on the inside. I loved George so much I didn't even mind that he began keeping those supermodels around as a way to deflect attention away from something, because I was still too young to know what he was trying to deflect attention from. I could hardly blame him for wanting to surround himself with beautiful women. Their presence didn't bother me at all. It just added a layer of titillation to our relationship that I didn't quite understand at the time.

As I got older, however, I realized I needed to get serious about my love interests. It was time to find a man who could devote himself to a purpose that was higher than simple entertainment, someone who was in pursuit of perfection. I set my sights on Olympic diver Greg Louganis. Maybe it was that million-dollar smile or all of the gold hardware around his neck—something about him was irresistible. While all of my boyfriends had each been different in key ways, they were remarkably similar, similar enough that I began to realize I had developed a type: Obviously, I was drawn to foreign men. I jest, naturally. Greg Louganis is clearly American.

Gay men have always held sway over me. I am drawn to them to this day. As a young girl, I think I instinctively knew there was something special about them, that maybe they held the secret to getting all I could ever want in a long-term relationship, things like companionship, a stylish house, and —most importantly—all of the sex on the side.

My husband hates that joke, probably because there's at least some truth to it.

This is not to say that I don't enjoy my monogamous marriage—I do. And I'm sure Chad would appreciate me mentioning that our intimate life is perfectly satisfying, but as time wears on, I can feel my sense of possessiveness over him dulling to a blunt tip. Whenever I hear that Carrie

Underwood song "Before He Cheats," I just feel exhausted for the poor girl who's wasting so much energy trashing her boyfriend's car while he's cozying up to some other gal at the pool hall.

"Just see it as one less thing on your to-do list, honey," I'll sigh to the radio before switching the station.

As a co-worker once told me while we were out at a bar one weekend with friends, there are a hundred things to love about being married. . .it was just the sex with one person that was his sticking point. I was young and single at the time, most likely a bit tipsy, and I remember swatting him on the arm and saying something inane like "Oh, Rob! You're so bad!" and letting him buy me another drink. Years later, when recounting this story to my husband, he just laughed at me.

"You know that he was trying to sleep with you, right?"

I could only blink at him as if I'd gone mute. It had never occurred to me that Rob might have been probing to see if I had the moral flexibility to sleep with a married man. I was simultaneously flattered and repulsed. And then flattered.

Nearly two decades into my own marriage now, I can understand my old co-worker's point. There are, indeed, a multitude of things that I love about being married, and sex is only one of them. I'm sure I could forgive most any indiscretion given this balance, and I doubt I could even be married to a man who is out of town more days than he is home if the possibility of infidelity always threatened to unwind me. It's a passiveness most of my female friends have a hard time understanding.

"Don't you worry about what he's doing while he's out on the road?" a neighbor once asked, seemingly unable to believe me when I insisted that I do not. Sure, every now and then Chad will come home with a new move in the bedroom, and I'll briefly wonder if he learned it from an accommodating flight attendant, but truth be told, I'm usually only curious because I'd like to know how to address the thank-you note.

Cheating is rarely strictly *personal*, it seems to me. That is, I believe I would see it as less of a rejection of me than it would be a signal that I am failing to provide something for my partner. Affairs usually stem from emotional need—it's almost never the sex that people are after when the final accounting is done. Or maybe it is. Maybe they just have a specific kink that their partner isn't into. I know I'd be happy to outsource any number of sexual perversions as long as the other woman agreed to take on camping duties, too.

My colleague who was educating me on the joys and trials of marriage all those years ago was about the age that I am now, so I have become more sympathetic to the predicament he found himself in. As my own mid-life crisis bears down, reminding me that my years as a desirable sexual being are drawing to a close, I can certainly understand the temptation to seek out one last thrill. Who wouldn't want to feel wanted again, rather than needed or—worse yet—simply available? This waning sense of vitality can be a real threat to a marriage, cliché as it may be.

Chad and I have begun to notice that people who struggle at this point in their relationship often take up "running" with an attractive friend. The more free-spirited types we know have tried out alternative lifestyles for a while. The very idea of this shocked me at first, but it's becoming so commonplace that whenever I see a proposal story hit the news, I think to myself *This is sweet and all, but I'd really like to see this couple twenty years from now, when one of them is proposing an open marriage. Now that would be good television.*

~

My husband and I are lucky to have a relatively uncomplicated marriage, and monogamy seems perfectly agreeable to us so far. But we're practically newlyweds in pilot years, considering we've only ever lived together about 50% of the time. Chad was on active duty in the Air Force when we first met, flying two and three-week sorties abroad with breaks of a few days to a few weeks in between before moving to the airlines later in life, ensuring that he was out of the house at least three nights a week. Since I was an only child who was used to spending a lot of time alone, this arrangement suited me just fine. More than fine, actually. The space was something of a necessity.

Whenever Chad is home for too long, I'll playfully feed him this same line: *Why don't you give me a chance to miss you.* Embedded in that request is also the converse: *Give yourself a little break from me,* which I try to throw in every now and then as a tacit acknowledgement that I'm a nightmare to live with.

We had figured out, years before Ester Perel burst onto the self-help scene with her book *Mating in Captivity,* that some amount of distance is necessary for the health of any long-term relationship. Perel's book outlines how couples doom themselves to a life without desire because they attempt to be everything to one another—best friend, lover, confidante. . .name the role. Modern marriage demands this kind of intimacy, but desire requires space. In our efforts to cultivate a sense of oneness, we kill any chance of *wanting* one another. It's a tale as old as time. My sexually frustrated former co-worker could attest to the truth of it.

There had always been enough space in my marriage to keep the home fires burning so to speak, so I didn't have much use for Perel's book. A sex advice column I'm fond of reading was always mentioning it, so I decided on a whim to buy it.

Chad and I share an e-book library, and he noticed my purchase while he was on a trip. He began reading it out of curiosity and finished it in utter panic before returning home, eager to discuss it with me. He was prepared with examples of women who loved their husbands but were un-satisfied because they were addicted to the limerent phase of a relationship, that time when sparks are flying and you're desperate enough for each other to agree to have sex in a car, a phase we had, admittedly, long grown out of. Plus, he suspected that my old sex-on-the-side line was more than innocent joking, and he wanted to know what he could do to keep me interested. I found his earnestness endearing. The secret was so simple.

"Just stay away from me as much as possible," I said before kissing him.

It truly is that easy. Who needs the complication of an open marriage to keep things fresh? Distance alone is a mir-acle cure for any relationship. No matter what quarrels Chad and I might have with one another or how much we might be getting under each other's skin, the moment he leaves for a trip, I begin to miss him. Twenty-four hours later, I will actually crave his presence. I'll even begin to wonder if my gay husband and I really would have had it so good. We'd probably wind up having the same taste in men, which would be a disaster for us both, because I'm incredibly competitive.

By the time Chad returns, I'm eager enough for a reunion, and he'll leave again before I even have the chance to wonder how a bald man can leave so much hair in the bathroom sink.

We live an awfully long time these days, and the prospect of spending that lifetime sharing space with a person who knows how to push all of your buttons can feel daunting. This is why I find it ideal to be married to a traveling man. Our part-time arrangement keeps the daily annoyances from piling up, which, in turn, keeps our tenderness for each other intact. This is not to say that everyone should marry a pilot, but the relationship certainly comes with perks beyond all the free flying. When time together is in short supply, it's far easier to remember to push the right buttons for each other every now then. And pilots, of all people, are very skilled at following a checklist.

8

The AI in Anxiety

New tech keeps appearing in my house. I assume my husband is responsible for this trend, but I've watched enough *Black Mirror* to be convinced that the tech might just be multiplying on its own. Most of it I could live without. The voice-controlled lights and the sous vide that's hooked up to my phone are nice, but they're a touch on the side of excess in my opinion. Our Google Home device occupies some nebulous middle ground. I was irritated when Chad brought one home a few years back without consulting me, but all was forgiven when I realized I finally had something in the house that would listen to everything I said. I decided it could stay.

The Google Home will rattle off a list of your appointments, update you on traffic conditions and the weather, and read you the news the moment you tell it "Good morning!" Since I work from home, it mostly just reminds me that I have a mid-afternoon appointment to cry alone in my bathroom and then asks if I would like it to schedule a tele-health visit with a therapist.

It's become something of a plaything for me, easily enter-tained as I am. I have trained my Google Home device to recognize my voice, and in turn, I have set a distinct voice to respond to me. I like having not just a personal assistant but a *personalized* one so that every time it speaks to me, it feels like I have a special relationship with technology that the rest of my family does not. For a while I had it speak to me in an Australian accent, but over time the novelty wore off, and I had to face the fact that I don't fully understand the metric system.

My husband has programmed a few shortcuts into the device, more for fun than convenience. For example, when I go to press my coffee in the morning, I need only say, "Cof-fee!" and my assistant will set a timer for one minute. This shortcut has winnowed down an eight-syllable request for a timer into a two-syllable command, which doesn't make me more productive necessarily, but it makes me feel heady with power, like a benevolent dictator, and gets me six syllables closer to my coffee.

Some mornings, when my voice is still gravelly with sleep, my assistant will not recognize me, and the default voice will answer. I usually respond with a forceful *Don't you know who I am?* before yelling something like *Bring back my regular girl!* There are obvious dangers to this kind of absolute power.

At some point in the last year, our original Google Home multiplied into something that I believe is called a Nest. There is now a device in nearly every room, helpfully boosting the wi-fi while listening in on all of our conversations.

Having so many devices in the house tends to create more chaos than convenience. When I commanded my assistant to set my coffee timer this morning, the dining room device answered me, which wouldn't normally be an issue except that, given the distance between us, it misheard my request and thought I had asked to call someone. While she was giving a lengthy lecture about how I hadn't set my account up to perform that task, I set another timer on the kitchen device. Meanwhile, the dining room's lecture had concluded, and it began calling someone. At 5:30 in the morning.

I panicked and began yelling at Google to hang up, but none of my commands were working—not cancel, not stop, not just hang up you *sonofabitch*—the ringing continued. I may have been forgetting to say "Hey Google" beforehand, like a Jeopardy contestant who had failed to phrase her answer in the form of a question, and I was being punished accordingly. When I finally got a response from the command "cancel everything," the kitchen Google answered that all timers and alarms would be stopped. But the ringing continued on. I finally ran over to the dining room device to turn it off manually and took a wild guess at when my coffee might have been finished steeping.

I still have no idea who Google was calling. This independent streak of hers is just beginning to trouble me.

More troubling than this independent streak, however, is the fact that I've been unconsciously referring to the device with female pronouns, as if there were actually a tiny woman being held hostage inside and forced to do my bidding. This tendency to anthropomorphize inanimate objects is a uniquely human trait, one that helps us to understand and empathize with others. It's admirable, but it seems fraught, too. When my children set an alarm for one hundred years in the future, which the device of course agreed to do, I became physically upset. I couldn't stomach the thought of this little machine sitting on a shelf somewhere, all of its masters long dead and gone, mournfully beeping into the void. That's a lot of emotion for something that most likely will kill me some day.

For now, in these halcyon days before the robot revolution, I am content to have her amuse me. Early on, I discovered that she had some charming quirks—a quality that only endeared her more to me—and among the more entertaining ones was her pronunciation of rap song titles. Since my family subscribes to Google's music service, we have access to nearly all of the music ever made simply by commanding the assistant to play whatever strikes our fancy. So when my husband got an itch to listen to the old Bone Thugs-n-Harmony song "For the Love of Money," his assistant happily complied.

"Sure. Now playing "Foe tha love of dollar sign," she said. She was not incorrect—that is exactly how the title was written—but still, we mocked her heartily and spent the next few minutes discovering other fun titles for our robot to mangle.

What's mildly disconcerting about this technology is that, within an hour of ridiculing her pronunciation of rap song titles, she had adopted our own pronunciations, reflecting not the literal data that she was collecting and relaying to us, but instead reflecting our white, middle-class, suburban interpretation of that information. Plenty could be extrapolated from that. Google has clearly hatched a plan for world domination, using every search and demand to power the engine of its god-machine in the cloud, and I can't help but wonder what, exactly, we're teaching it. Perhaps more importantly, which voices will predominantly do the teaching? Like the nuns who spent years "curing" a generation of school children of their left-handedness with the smack of a ruler, I managed to "cure" my assistant's speech patterns within an hour. That's an alarmingly fast learning curve.

What will eventually happen with all of this data is well beyond my ken, so I'll leave the problem in the hands of more capable social scientists. The world at large has become an all-consuming data collection machine, and there's just no stopping the march of progress. I'm not about to give up my assistant in protest. She's gotten to know me too well over the years, possibly because her Google overlords have programmed her to eavesdrop on me at all hours of the day. She thinks I don't know, but every now and then, she'll light up for no reason and I'll know that she's listening in. I figure she's lonely, so I really don't mind. In fact, I suspect she's listening in right now, from the device that's perched on a credenza in my office, a device I could swear was not there just yesterday.

9

Life is but a Dream

I posed a thought problem to my son: "Imagine the life you are living is merely a dream that another version of yourself—the *real you* if you will—is having. Every night, when the real you goes to sleep, it dreams your entire life in one night. Dream-you is a sentient being who believes that his world and life are real. When dream-you reaches the end of his life, he is simply reborn into the next night's dream. By the time the real you is also fourteen," I said, "the dream you would have already lived thousands of lifetimes."

Dylan furrowed his brow and looked uncomfortable with this line of thinking, but he was trapped in the car with no means of escape, which I have always found to be the best way to engage in conversation with children.

"Please stop," he begged. "You're making my head hurt."

I was already deep into this rabbit hole though, so there was no stopping me just yet.

"Then what if *dream-you* could *also* give birth to new lives every night in *his* sleep," I continued. "Your dream lives would expand exponentially!"

I was getting excited over the possibilities of my scenario, but I could hear my son groaning from the passenger seat, so I paused the mental torture and apologized.

"Thank you," he sighed, his body relaxing into the seat. "Why do you even like thinking about these crazy things?"

I drummed my fingers on the steering wheel as I considered his question.

"I guess I don't want to get too comfortable with what I think I know," I said.

~

I'm hardly alone in thinking these kinds of thoughts, though I'm probably one of the few who thinks them while stone sober. The nature of reality has always preoccupied philosophers and poets and people who just need a few hours of good sleep the night before an important meeting. In the 17th century, René Descartes proposed a thought problem in which he imagined an "evil demon" had crafted an illusory world designed to deceive him into trusting his senses as a way to understand the nature of reality:

"I shall think that the sky, the air, the earth, colours, shapes, sounds and all external things are merely the delusions of dreams which he has devised to ensnare my judgement," Descartes wrote. "I shall consider myself as not having hands or eyes, or flesh, or blood or senses, but as falsely believing that I have all these things."

The popular version of this line of questioning nowadays is to suppose that we're living in a computer simulation à la

The Matrix. Had Descartes lived in the 21ˢᵗ century, his "evil demon" would obviously be Google. Or Facebook.

The other day, my husband and I were kicking around the idea that this life of ours *could* be a simulation. It was the only way to make sense of what was happening in the world in COVID times: Either our programmers are toying with us, or they've implemented some kind of internship program that, needless to say, is not going well.

We went rounds about it for a while before putting the issue to bed, since it was impossible to arrive at any real answer. Not long after our conversation, my news aggregating app suggested I read a *Scientific American* article titled, "Do We Live in a Simulation? Chances are About 50-50."

"Look," I said to Chad, waving my phone in his face. The article prompted no response.

"Don't you remember our conversation? From yesterday?"

"Sure. So?"

"So? IT MEANS WE'RE DEFINITELY LIVING IN A SIMULATION!" I yelled.

He calmly took a sip of his coffee. "Or it means that Google really is listening all of the time."

~

I don't know that I actually believe the simulation hypothesis, nor does it really matter to me if it's true. Unless I can have access to the actual reality—"base" reality as it's come to be known—there's not much sense in fretting about it. But every now and then I'll have an experience that makes me question the fundamental nature of reality and consciousness, and I'll find myself unable to shake the feeling that things aren't quite what they may seem.

Shortly after my father died a few years ago, I began having dissociative episodes that left me with a persistent feeling that nothing was real. I was becoming convinced that my life was part of some kind of elaborate scheme, like the realistic dream state induced by Descartes' "evil demon." Sometimes I'd even take comfort in the thought that my father and I were living another version of this life somewhere, either in one of the dreams I proposed in the thought problem to my son, or on a planet exactly like our own, with exact replicas of us living our exact lives—a certainty if the universe, or multiverse as it were, is indeed infinite.

Most of this thinking could probably be attributed to the stress of losing a parent under challenging circumstances— my father had died from complications of a suicide attempt, and I was coming undone by it. But in the process of reflecting on my life with him, old memories resurfaced with such force and clarity, so vividly *alive*, I could convince myself that our former lives were still happening, our younger selves intact, permanently fixed somewhere along the space-time continuum.

There's an idea that supposes all of existence, everything that is, was, or ever will be, has already been etched into some cosmic DVD, and our consciousness is the machine that allows us to watch the movie (I'm paraphrasing), creating an illusion that time is linear. This is known as the Static Theory of Time. To me, the immediacy and vibrance of those old memories made a compelling emotional case for this theory, and I began to reflect on other times I'd encountered this feeling in my life, as if to compile more evidence in support of this static view of the universe.

Shortly after my college graduation, I was walking down the street on a placid afternoon in Syracuse, when something in a tree branch caught my eye. I stopped walking and stared at the rustling leaves. The breeze picked up, and in its rush, the real world fell away. I was nearly knocked sideways by an overwhelming feeling that my sense of time, maybe even my sense of existence, had been all wrong. For a brief moment, I believed I was physically feeling everything I had ever experienced and everything I *would come to* experience in my life—all of the joy and sorrow, the sensations of being born, living, and dying. It all washed over me in a disorienting tidal wave before receding into whatever metaphysical sea had spawned it. I stumbled to the front stoop of a friend's house and sat there for a few minutes, dazed. For years I tried to characterize what had happened to me—one part near-death experience, one part awakening—but I could never find a way to convey the magnitude of what had occurred. No one seemed to understand my experience, which only amplified its sense of importance. I felt anointed.

It may have been nothing—a simple case of vertigo or mild dehydration from too much indulging the night before. But I was facing several radical life changes at the time—leaving the cocoon of college to enter the military at a post overseas was foremost on my mind—and the anxiety about these changes likely prompted what is known in the medical parlance as *derealization* and *depersonalization.*

People with anxiety disorders tend to have this type of experience as a fairly routine response to stress, but anyone under extreme duress might have one from time to time. In depersonalization, people sometimes report having "out of body" experiences or changes to their perceptions of reality. Derealization can create distortions in the appearance of the environment or in the perception of time. As soon as I learned these terms, I finally understood the pathology of my old-memory moments and my mystical experience with the Syracuse trees. I was crushed.

For twenty-odd years I had gone through life thinking I'd had a profound spiritual awakening, had maybe even been given the key to unlocking the mysteries of time and reality, likely because those endless nights I spent in my childhood learning how to astral project put me on a different spiritual plane than everyone else. Instead, I discovered that my brain was just stressed out. So much for being exceptional. And as I thought more about this experience through the years, I realized I had been suffering from these perfectly normal, scientifically explainable episodes for most of my life.

I began having depersonalization events when I was a young child, perhaps five or six years old. One day, I was standing in front of the open refrigerator, looking at the condiments that were stuffed into the door, when I had the distinct sense that my consciousness had separated from my body. It wasn't that I felt I was outside of my body watching myself as I looked into the refrigerator—I was aware that I was seeing through my own eyes and feeling the cool air on my skin. Kinesthetically, I was still operating normally. But my consciousness—or what I think of as consciousness, anyway— had become an internal observer of what was happening with my body, as if it were some other entity trapped inside.

The feeling was so arresting that I felt my legs begin to soften with fear, and I began trying to talk myself back into my body. "You are Joanna," I said to myself. "You are getting mayonnaise from the refrigerator. That is your hand. This is your body."

The episodes, when they do still occur, happen in much the same way: dissociation, followed by a brief panic, then negotiation. The negotiation piece turned out to be the most important part of the process and the one that kept me from entering a graveyard spiral of anxiety about the anxiety itself. The most commonly accepted way of ending this kind of stress response is to calmly and rationally talk yourself back into your body. I somehow knew this instinctively as a child, so maybe there's still room for some belief in my exceptionalism.

Sometimes I wonder what would happen if I couldn't forge a truce between my body and my consciousness when this happens, if I'm not simply anxious but teetering on the edge of madness. But what is madness but a disconnect between our internal and external lives? If we can't say for certain that there's an objective reality, that we're not the products of an evil demon's dream, how can we evaluate anyone's sanity? This both troubles and relieves me.

I think back to that conversation with my son, the one with the silly thought problem about dream lives. I had told him that I pose these problems to myself so that I don't get complacent about what I think I know, but that's really not it at all. I already suspected that I know nothing. The thought problems only confirm it.

10

Finding Your Voice

The voice inside my head, the one that provides near constant narration of my day-to-day tasks and occasionally answers me when I talk to myself, is British. I don't know why this is. I never really noticed this until the other day, when I was carrying a paper-wrapped bundle under my arm, the little voice piped up in a cross between Mary Poppins and Mrs. Doubtfire and said, "My! My parcels are so cumbersome!"

I don't ever utter the word "parcels" in real life. The word exists only in my head when this Briton of vague pedigree is talking. I'm not sure who she is. I do have a good chunk of British ancestry, so maybe she's a long-dead relative who's managed to live on as a voice inside my head, like some pre-digital-age consciousness transplant. But I imagine she's still me, just a jauntier version.

Once upon a time, making a confession like this would have gotten me branded as a witch and burned or tossed into an asylum, depending on the century. Nowadays it might get me a Twitter following. Times have changed—mostly for the better.

Still, quirks like this that so much as hint at mental illness tend to give me pause. I was born with a bit of faulty wiring in my brain that sparks in relatively minor ways on occasion, but I can't help but wonder what would happen if one of those sparks set off a full-blown fire. I wouldn't be the first woman in my family to go down in these metaphorical flames.

According to family legend, my fifth great-grandmother, Elizabeth Buttermore Harshman, was involuntarily committed to a Pennsylvania mental institution by her husband George, who claimed she was a danger to herself and her community. It's hard to say what, exactly, her condition might have been—women at the time could be committed simply for having strong opinions or moods—but I've always felt an affinity for her because of this fate.

In 1852, the year this was alleged to have happened, Elizabeth would have just given birth to her 12th child, a boy named Franklin Pierce. Her first child had arrived in 1836, when she was just a young woman of 20 tending the land alongside her husband, and she found that a child came along reliably every one to two years until Franklin. Between the demands of caring for young children and working a farm, it's difficult to imagine how she and George found time to make so many children in the first place. But producing a steady supply of farm hands was part of Elizabeth's job description at the time, and she did what was expected of her. . .until she apparently just couldn't.

For whatever reason, her story had stuck with me ever

since I read about it on an Ancestry.com message board nearly a decade ago. Then one day, out of the blue, I found that I *had* to know more about what prompted her committal, so I took a quick trip to Pennsylvania to spend a few days in the Fayette County Courthouse looking for the court documents that would have proven this story to be true. This might seem an absurd thing to do, to fly across the country to retrieve something that could be entirely made up, but as an airline spouse flying costs me nothing, and my mother was available to meet me for part of the trip, so the enterprise wasn't completely loony. Nevertheless, it's probably not most women's idea of a fun getaway.

I had high hopes going into the project, particularly since the message board post that had initially piqued my interest included an update indicating that a researcher in Fayette County had found the documents that would confirm the story. It was an old message with no way to contact the original poster, so until I could get my hands on the papers myself, the story was still just that—a story. But at least I had a lead.

I arrived in Pennsylvania in the early evening and settled into my cabin about a half hour outside of Uniontown, at a secluded country estate called Fernstone Retreat. Fernstone's pastoral setting made it an ideal place for weddings, but individual cabins were rented out whenever an event wasn't scheduled. I elected to stay in the Tree House, which I might have avoided had I noticed beforehand that it was usually used by newlyweds, but I decided to just embrace the energy of the place and took to calling it the "conjugal suite" until my mother joined me there the next day and asked me to stop.

I set off for the court house on that first morning the most rested person ever to emerge from the conjugal suite, and I happily locked myself away in a dusty attic records repository, combing through boxes of documents that were so old and fragile I often feared they might crumble in my hands. In an office below, a city employee was making phone calls to other government offices, eager to help me narrow my search. I'd never met a more pleasant and accommodating government employee.

Unfortunately, despite hours of diligent work, my search turned up nothing. I stored my paperwork in my rental car and took note of an evangelical group that had gathered on the courthouse steps to publicly pray for President Trump. I certainly wasn't in the Pacific Northwest anymore.

I walked around downtown Uniontown for a bit, admiring the architecture and trying to situate myself in the place through time, to see it through the eyes of my ancestors. Certain lines of my family had lived their entire lives in the confines of the county, often times only venturing off when they answered the call to serve during wartime, and of course that was only the men. Many of the women, most in fact, went from their father's house to their husband's house, and —if they hadn't married well—to the poor house with little say in the matters. Such an insular life could drive anyone to madness, twelve children or not. I didn't need a court document to understand how poor Eliza might have landed in the asylum.

It's lucky I had come to this conclusion, because just as I was mulling over the next steps for my research, my phone rang with bad news. It was the city employee who had been helping me find the records I was looking for. The tone of her voice seemed genuinely sympathetic. My heart sank.

"I'm sorry to tell you this," she said, "but it looks like the batch of records you're looking for was being stored off-site in a church attic, and they were destroyed by pigeons a few years ago."

I let out a little snort. "I'm sorry. Did you say *pigeons*?"

I had no doubt that Elizabeth's husband George had a hand in this. It would seem fitting for him to have been reincarnated as a pigeon, considering how he treated his poor wife all those years ago. Just after her disappearance, he pawned baby Franklin off onto his oldest daughter, then moved with one of his sons to Iowa, where he almost immediately remarried. Coming back as a pigeon after that is the kind of karma that really makes sense to me.

But as a pigeon, defecating all over the records was all he needed to do to cover his tracks, and now no one will ever know what really transpired between the couple. The asylum story might very well have been made up. But the fact that it coincides with the birth of their last child suggests that Elizabeth might have been suffering from post-partum depression or maybe even post-partum psychosis—either would have been inexplicable and frightening for everyone at the time. She needed help when help was not available. She needed to be a voice for her children, who still needed a mother. And she needed a voice for herself when the culture—and the law —had rendered her mute.

No matter the truth of Elizabeth's story, she certainly never had the opportunity to experience a fully actualized life, tethered as she was to the farm and her family. But I have to stop myself from feeling sorry for my foremothers, even though their suffering is clearly worthy of my sympathy. I have to remind myself that they live on through me, through the genes that have been passed onto me through time. While their lives may have been insular, mine has been expansive. I have travelled the world alone. I own property. I see a therapist without the threat of being committed to a mental institution by my husband.

While my foremothers were voiceless, I have a pen and paper and an audience and an impact. By extension, they do, too. I'm proud of their legacy that I am carrying forward. And while I can't speak for all of my foremothers, I feel confident in speaking for Elizabeth when I say that George deserved to come back as something much lower than a pigeon.

II

An Essay Concerning
Avian Understanding

My daughter and I were walking home from the grocery store when we saw two birds, apparently pigeons, fall from the eaves of a nearby house and into the grass, engaged in some kind of scuffle. To be more accurate, it appeared that a few crows had flushed the pigeons out of the eaves and then hung out nearby, squawking like they were encouraging a schoolyard fight.

There was something off in how the pigeons were interacting. The one underneath was frantically beating its wing, which prompted me to wonder aloud if we were witnessing an unwelcomed mating attempt. As Rowan and I inched closer, however, I could see that the top pigeon was not a pigeon at all but some kind of small hawk, either a Cooper's or a sharp-shinned—I couldn't be sure. It's not uncommon to see small raptors in the city, as they're keen enough to make hunting grounds of the areas around bird feeders, but it was at the very least unexpected to see this hawk attacking a bird its own size if not slightly larger. At any rate, once we knew what we were looking at, we realized we were witnessing a murder-in-progress, and we obviously stopped everything to take it all in. We're always up for quality time together.

This was not the first time Rowan and I had seen a hawk attack. A few years ago, one was coolly draining the life out of a Northern Flicker in our front yard, and we watched the scene unfold from our living room window. Rowan was enthralled.

"This is so *entertaining*," she said more than once, which I noted with a hint of concern before returning to the window with a bag of popcorn. In that case, the flicker managed to escape, hiding in the wheel well of our neighbor's truck until the hawk eventually abandoned the chase.

The pigeon, however, was not as lucky. As we approached, the hawk flew off to join the gang of crows on some power lines hanging just overhead, but when the dazed pigeon began to rouse itself, the crows swooped in again, providing a diversion while the hawk dove down to sink its talons into its victim one final time. I can't say that I delighted in the spectacle, but the crows' involvement intrigued me. They seemed to be working *with* the hawk in taking down this hapless pigeon. It was like watching Churchill and Roosevelt ally themselves with Stalin. None of it made any sense. Crows and hawks generally have an adversarial relationship, not a cooperative one. It could be that I was misinterpreting what was happening, that the crows were actually mobbing the hawk, but that would have meant that they were defending the pigeon, which also would have made no sense. I'm still at a loss for how to explain what was happening.

Unlikely as this alliance might have been, it wouldn't be the strangest relationship the natural world has ever seen. I recently read about an orca whale dubbed "Old Tom," who spent decades helping Australian fishermen catch baleen whales. Old Tom and his pod would trap the whales in a shallow bay then alert the fishermen by slapping the water. Once the baleen whales had been killed, the orcas would feed on their lips and tongues, leaving the valuable blubber for the fishermen. The whaling family that developed this relationship with the orcas called this phenomenon the "Law of the Tongue," and observed it for three generations before Old Tom died and his pod either abandoned the area or was hunted out of existence.

I'm not suggesting that cooperation between two different species of birds is quite as remarkable as this relationship between humans and whales, but I'm trying to make room for the possibility that communication—maybe even *understanding*—can happen, even in unlikely places. This idea might be more inspiring if the animals in my example had not come together to form an understanding about murder, but nature is brutal, and everyone has to eat.

Had the universe seen fit to show me a mother cat nursing an orphaned squirrel, I probably would have been moved to write about these strange alliances from a much more uplifting angle. But it didn't. It showed me death and the thrill of the hunt, and I am trying to find something if not necessarily beautiful then at least harmonious in these displays of cooperation, proof that nature synthesizes and connects in ways that speak to some fundamental truth. I haven't quite landed on what I believe that truth to be. Maybe that's the work of our lives, to come to some awareness of this interconnectedness.

When the scuffle was over between the pigeon and the hawk, the crows quieted, surveying the scene from their perch on the power lines, waiting to see what could be scavenged. I took my daughter's hand, felt her fingers slip neatly between my own.

"Maybe the hawk will leave them something," I said. "As a kind of payment for their help."

"The crows can always find something, Mom," she said before adding, almost as an afterthought, "They're happy with the things no one else wants."

12

Want Not

I'm inclined to wax nostalgic about *The Wizard of Oz*, specifically about how I used to delight in the anticipation of seeing something that only came around once a year, with all of the related fanfare of such an event. People would talk about it for days—perhaps weeks—before it aired, and I remember the lead-up being almost on par with Christmas in terms of excitement. As much as waiting for anything was insufferable to me as a child, the process of waiting for *The Wizard of Oz* each year taught me that the anticipation of a thing could be nearly as satisfying as the thing itself. I would come to appreciate the nuances of this idea later in life, but at five years old, it was only ruby slippers that I waited for and coveted.

Today, it's hard to understand how watching a movie on television could produce such a thrill. We have become habit-uated to instant gratification in ways that are obvious enough: Our entertainment is consumed on demand. Arguments are settled and curiosities satisfied with an internet search rather than a trip to the library. Even a date can be summoned with the casual swipe of a finger. We wait for precious little.

So, when the podcast *Serial* began airing a few years ago, releasing a new episode each Thursday, I found that, for the first time in many years, I could revisit the pleasures of waiting for some simple thing. This particular kind of joy-in-anticipation was shared collectively on social media, where #IsItThursdayYet became the hashtag emblem of our weekly wait, likely created by a person who never learned patience by trying to tape record a song from the radio.

All of this must have been too much for the younger crowd to bear, because when *Serial* created the spin-off *S-Town*, the show was released all at once in "binge-worthy" fashion. This disappointed me, as I had not only appreciated the space for contemplation the time between episodes had given me, I had also enjoyed, to some extent, the shared "suffering" of waiting with other fans. There is communion in adversity, however slight the shared trials might be.

I tried to manufacture a sense of anticipation for the new show by restricting myself to an episode a week, but as anyone who has tried to resist eating cookies by hiding them knows—well, you just always know where the cookies are hiding. The temptation to binge was too great and chatter about the show was all around me. I eventually succumbed and listened to the whole series at once, though all I really wanted was some quiet time to think on some things—the desperation of a closeted life in the South, for example, or the isolation and despair in the life of an eccentric genius. I wanted to think and talk about poverty and humanity. In truth, I could have even spent an afternoon thinking about mottos inscribed on sundials: *Serius est quam cogitas:* It's later than you think. *Tempus breve est:* Time is short.

Time is short. Indeed, we know. Perhaps that is the impetus behind our impulse to seek out pleasure in the moment, to seize the day as Horace decreed: *Carpe diem, quam minimum credula postero.*

Seize the day, trusting little in tomorrow.

This could be the motto for our modern time. I recently asked an older colleague if he thought this instant and abundant gratification was detrimental to our happiness. He smiled at me in a fatherly way, his head at a tilt as if amused by my question.

"Yes," he said without further explication.

"What are we supposed to DO about it then," I nearly yelled, pounding my fists on the desk between us.

Apparently, I expected wisdom on demand along with everything else.

~

When I first set out to write this, I thought I was going to explore what is lost when our every whim is satisfied at any time, when we lose our capacity to find some measure of joy in waiting. I didn't care to get into the Big Ideas here, ones about striving and sacrificing for noble things; I wanted to know, more than anything, how I could recapture that feeling from my youth, that anticipation for something that was, but for one day a year, being denied me. But that is not where I am being led.

In his *Discourses*, the Stoic philosopher Epictetus highlights the pitfalls of the very thing I had set out to defend and reclaim, though what I had framed as anticipation he had named desire: "It's not only the desire for wealth and position that debases and subjugates us, but also the drive for peace, leisure, travel, and learning. It doesn't matter what the external thing is, the value we place on it subjugates us to another. . .where our heart is set, there our impediment lies."

Anticipation of any kind, he argues, makes us a slave to the objects of those desires. It interferes with our ability to live in the moment, savoring what is actually in our midst. We are never present, only wanting.

It seems I've been asking the wrong questions all along. It is wanting that is the *problem*, not the reward. Rather than ask how to recapture that innocent excitement, I should have been asking, *How can I curb my desires in the first place?* This is a thornier problem. From clever marketing to social media influencers, the culture largely tells us what we should want. I would have been pleased to watch *The Wizard of Oz* with my family had it simply happened to be on, but I spent a week or more obsessing over the show precisely because the network and its advertisers had built an obsessive hype around it. This tactic is powerful enough that now, four decades later, I still fall victim to this manufactured desire, still *want the wanting* of the next thing someone tells me to consume.

There is a contraction of the contemplative space when we constantly, casually consume, whether it's entertainment or news or cheap goods from the developing world that we're swallowing wholesale. There's simply no space for reflection on the meaning or value of any of it. That, in the end, is what I've really been missing—the space. Desire was merely a distraction.

Still, I feel compelled to reflect on the value of the things that bring me joy. I do want that feeling after all, even if I want to be freed from the desire preceding it. As I began toying with this idea, I made a list of ordinary things I look forward to and queried a few friends for ideas of their own. Our lists were remarkably similar. We look forward to food, mainly, to plump June strawberries and the first sweet corn of summer. We look forward to things the natural world offers us—a sunny day in winter or the first warm blush of spring, the abrupt arrival of fall, its air cutting like a knife's edge. We look forward to a real conversation amid a sea of idle chatter.

But we love each thing in its season, accepting it as it arrives, on a timeline set by forces wholly out of our control. There is no real yearning for these things, merely delight in their eventual arrival. I want to live my life mindful of this, to accept these gifts as they present themselves, not as I might hope for them in a future that may never be. After all, it is later than I think.

13

Involuntary Napping and Other Afflictions

I had been awake for about three hours when I took my first nap of the day. It was a Saturday, with nothing on the schedule by design, and my husband and I had just walked home from breakfast. I had slept well the night before and hadn't felt particularly fatigued while we were out, but the minute we returned, I was so overcome by sleepiness that I flopped onto the couch and passed out without a care. I woke up maybe twenty minutes later, stretching like a cat, saying—in a thick Southern accent that must have been lingering in my brain from watching Fortune Feimster the night before—"I just took me a biscuits and gravy nap!"

I staggered off of the couch and went on about my day for approximately three more hours, at which point I noticed a rare ray of sunshine streaming through the front window. It called to me, and I couldn't resist lying down in it and falling asleep again, this time for several hours. When I woke from my second nap of the day, I figured I should hit the gym to boost my energy level a bit. But after stumbling up the stairs to change my clothes, I found my bed more enticing than the gym, and I decided it was necessary to "rest my eyes" from those taxing five minutes I had been employing them since my last nap. I only woke up when my husband called me down to dinner.

My third nap allowed me to get through dinner and half of an *Avengers* movie, which I would have slept through under most circumstances anyway, so my fourth nap wasn't much of a surprise. When the movie was over, I went to bed, exhausted from all of the napping, and slept as soundly as if I'd spent the day toiling in a coal mine.

It's fair to say that I've been mildly depressed. Maybe more than mildly. I likely spent all of Saturday sleeping because I had spent the previous few days crying my way through various things—books, meetings, movies—and I was just exhausted.

I thought I had been muddling through this low period in my own messy and imperfect way, just under the radar of people I interact with regularly, when a friend sat me down and asked how I was doing. The concern on his face was obvious.

"I'm fine," I insisted.

He raised an eyebrow. "Fine-fine, or *fucked-up, insecure, neurotic, and emotional* fine? Because people are worried about you."

I couldn't help but laugh at this, even as the tears welled up against my will. I had never heard this take on the word fine before, though a quick Google search revealed that it's been in use forever, and I wondered how it has escaped my attention all these years. The acronym suits me—well—just *fine* to be honest, even when I'm not depressed.

But I have been depressed these last several weeks. That I know. I have always been a melancholy person, easily moved to tears and given to brooding, and what I've learned about having such a personality is this: If you sit with your sadness for a moment, it can give you a measure of clarity and perspective. Sit with it for too long and it will consume you.

What began as a bit of wallowing during the anniversary of my father's death somehow morphed into an overwhelming existential crisis of sorts, leaving me to feel like some kind of two-dimensional black-and-white version of myself, devoid of any sense of passion or purpose. Some of this is typical middle-age ennui. Some of it is a deeper, more intractable problem of brain chemistry. Much of it is negative thinking left to run amok. All of it is draining.

I've gone rounds about how much to divulge here, mainly because I find that writing about depression is not therapeutic; it's another form of "sitting with my sadness," which only perpetuates the cycle of negative thinking and prolongs the period of depression. There's real work to be done to get through these episodes—being mindful, practicing gratitude, nourishing the physical body. Those parts tend to get lost in our culture of ease.

Still, I think it's worthwhile to share the simple fact that I'm struggling a bit, if only to let others who are going through similar challenges know that they are not alone. It can be all the more confounding to feel this way when life is objectively great. If I'm not careful, I can convince myself that feeling anything less than joyful gratitude for everything in my life is simply an invitation to real hardship. An anxiety spiral is never helpful to the recovery process. There is still gratitude, but there is also pain. They are not mutually exclusive.

I find it's much easier to write about anxiety, since it tends to manifest in more amusing ways. But I'm beginning to see some of the humor in how depression manifests as well, so I take that as a sign that things are looking up. My day of involuntary napping felt a bit like a fever breaking, the point during an illness when the body has finished its fight and, cool and rested, can turn its attention toward healing.

And I believe I can feel it—the healing. Yesterday was filled with sunshine and sweetbox and a visit from the dearest of old friends. Today, I felt the stirrings of some creative energy and wrote for a bit. I'm feeling hopeful, so I know I will be fine in time (while continuing to be F.I.N.E.). I might be even better after a little nap.

Station Break

Allow me to account for the recent sadness.

14

The Cruelest Month

I can connect
Nothing with nothing.
The broken fingernails of dirty hands.
My people humble people who expect
Nothing.
   – T.S. Eliot, from "The Wasteland"

Lately I've been drawn to visual representations of transitions, to paths that wend their way out of frame, for example, and to liminal spaces—the dusk mainly, where light and darkness submit to one another, each day sighing into night. I take note of shrouding fog, how it reduces the world to suggestion and abstraction, how I can look at the sun and mistake it for the moon. The ambiguity of this is wondrously disorienting. But everything eventually takes its form.

December is the cruelest month—apologies to Mr. Eliot. It is this month that seems to force me into these observations, to acknowledge that we are always standing at some unseen threshold, one shuddering breath from sighing into our own eternal night. Or, in the case of my father, 18 days spent slouching toward that darkness.

What do you call a suicide attempt that fails initially but later claims the person's life? A delayed suicide? Death from complications of a suicide attempt? Or simply an untimely death? Years later, I still don't know how to characterize how my father died. The call announcing his suicide attempt came on December 10th and the one announcing his death came on December 28th. In the interim, I swooped into my father's hospital room, offering promises that things could be different—a familiar tale he had always been fond of telling, even if it was a fiction.

Still, I asked the question: "Would you feel you had something to live for if I could get you to a place closer to me? If the kids and I could visit you regularly?"

He stared at his feet while he considered this. His guts, which he had ripped from his body days earlier, were contained in a silicone bag that rested on top of his abdomen. A nursing student the hospital had assigned to suicide watch stood behind him, listening in.

He shrugged his shoulders, never looking me in the eye. "Sure, I guess," he said.

I nodded. "Then I'll do my best to get you closer to me."

But things would never be different. That much we both knew. My father fell asleep shortly after this conversation, and I noted in his ragged breathing another liminal space, one he had taught me to recognize years earlier in roommates he would outlive at the veteran's home where he had been residing.

"You can hear death coming before you can see it," he had said.

~

Though I know my father had already resolved to die before I came barging in to play the role of some self-appointed savior, I am still haunted by our final conversation. Did my offer to help give him hope in his final days? And if so, was that hope a balm or a torment? When I am feeling uncharitable toward myself, I imagine the fear he might have felt had I given him reason to believe he did, in fact, want to live, only to realize he had already set into motion a series of events that could not be undone. I wake up in a cold sweat some nights dreaming of this.

I can only hope the reverse is true—that he died with the knowledge that his daughter loved him enough to fight on his behalf, that she still believed he could find something worth living for. That he could die with a sense of peace.

Though this guilt still gnaws at me, the grief has abated. I will still find joy in the holidays, even if they are tinged with a certain melancholy. That's all of life, though, isn't it? But December truly is the cruelest month. For now, I repeat certain lines of poetry like a prayer—*Shantih shantih shantih*—and hope that this peace is waiting for me at the threshold of the new year.

We now return to our regularly scheduled programming.

15

Captain Cook's Revenge

During a family vacation to Hawai'i, my husband and I took our kids to Kealakekua Bay to paddle to the spot where Captain Cook was killed by the native Hawaiians in the late 18th century. Because this is our family's idea of fun. It was a perfect morning, clear and cool. I surveyed the bay and declared it a beautiful place to die, then onto the water we went.

I generally don't mind being on the water, but I'm not fond of being *in* the water, particularly where carnivorous creatures are known to live. And this is without ever having seen the movie *Jaws*. So when my son jumped out of the kayak to snorkel, I was a bit on edge.

"You're sure there are no sharks in the bay," I whispered to my husband, who was sitting with our daughter on a paddleboard next to me. He just rolled his eyes at me. I knew this was meant to communicate *You're being ridiculous*, but his vague non-answer also left room for the possibility that there absolutely were sharks in the water. Because the universe enjoys toying with me, at that very moment, blood inexplicably began to gush from my daughter's nose and dripped into the water where her brother was swimming.

I don't believe there's a sensible way to have a panic attack of any kind, but there's certainly no sensible way to have a panic attack in a kayak while your child is actively bleeding into what you are now convinced are shark infested waters. I was immediately seized by a vision of some razor-toothed mouth emerging from the deep to drag my children below the surface as they clutched their snorkel gear to their chests, saying solemnly, "We only wanted to see the angelfish. . ."

Somehow I refrained from screaming, "YOU'RE ABOUT TO BE EATEN BY A SHARK!" and I calmly convinced my son to get out of the water so that we could get closer to the Cook monument. Tour boats were dumping snorkelers into the water in that direction, and I was certain the sharks would prefer to attack the boaters.

We paddled on without being eaten. In the shallows near the monument, both kids snorkeled successfully with their father while I hung back with the boats clenching my teeth. I briefly tried to see what was swimming around below me, but I only needed to stick my face in the water to bring about an episode of panicked gasping. I decided to be content with the children's occasional reports to me.

In the end, nothing was lurking below the surface but my anxiety, and even then it didn't pull me under, which was a significant victory for me. It's always there, lurking, like the shark that *did* attack a swimmer a few days later, just north of the bay where we were paddling. This is the flaw in anxiety: We're *always* swimming with sharks. Most days they don't attack. Some days they do. Captain Cook could tell you about how quickly tides can turn. It's a struggle to make peace with the inherent risks in life, but I do. I must. If I want to know more happiness than fear in life, I have to keep getting into the water.

16

The Doctor Will See You Now

I recently had a dermatologist look at something I'm fairly certain is skin cancer, though the patch of skin in question had unhelpfully healed just prior to my appointment. The doctor assured me that this is common enough, given the lag time between scheduling an appointment and actually being seen, and he handed me a mirror and a pen to have me point out the section of skin that concerned me. I took the pen and began drawing a large circle around the tip of my nose before I stopped and said, "Wait. Did you want me to use the pen as a pointer or to actually draw on my face?"

One guess which one he wanted.

For the next 15 minutes, I sat in the exam chair trying to appear thoughtful and serious as I listened to the doctor speak, all while the tip of my nose was outlined in a very prominent circle of blue ink. To add insult to injury, this doctor also happened to be quite handsome, which made me wish for a skin cancer that would at least kill me swiftly, if not instantly.

This kind of experience is fairly typical for me. I once broke out into a teary-eyed laughing fit while my dentist's hands were knuckle-deep in my mouth all because I'd overheard the hygienist in the next room ask her young patient if she could hold his balls. When that got no response, she helpfully suggested that he put them in his pocket. As the mother of a pre-teen boy at the time, it was all too much for me to bear.

But in my defense, I am not always the one perpetrating the awkwardness at my medical appointments. As a young woman, I had an Aussie doctor expose my breasts for an exam only to say, with an odd enthusiasm, "You'll never have any trouble examining those!"

I was too busy staring at the cat poster on the ceiling for her comment to fully register with me, but I must have muttered something like, "Wha—?" because she felt the need to continue.

"Oh, it's ok," she assured me. "Flat-chested women are far more intelligent!"

I might have taken offense, but her accent was both beguiling and somewhat unintelligible, so I just accepted that I had heard a compliment buried in what she was saying and thought to myself: *The doctor has spoken.* Then I silently praised my genes for investing more energy into my brain than my bust.

But that was twenty years ago. These days, there's something about being in a doctor's office that sends my IQ score plummeting, despite the intelligence conferred by my small breasts. Whenever I am handed a hospital gown, for example, I immediately forget the nurse's instructions and am left in a mild panic wondering which articles of clothing I am supposed to remove. My instinct, when handed a robe, is to completely undress. This would seem a reasonable assumption in most cases, but I stripped down for my last annual exam only to have the doctor arrive to tell me that yearly pelvic exams were a thing of the past. I tried to convince her that I had just wanted to air out a bit while I waited, but in truth, I simply expected to be uncomfortable and exposed in an exam room. It's part of the experience.

Then again, life is generally an uncomfortable experience for me. When I am not smearing ink on my face or stripping needlessly, I am still marked by my awkwardness, so plainly and painfully *exposed* most of the time. I've never been good at hiding my feelings or biting my tongue. I can get deeply personal with casual acquaintances. I tend to say the wrong things at the worst possible times. But if the Aussie doctor is any indication, we're all capable of acting like a boob from time to time, no matter how poised and gracious we might otherwise be.

Most people forgive me my quirkiness. Some even keep me around solely to bear witness to whatever buffoonery I might get into. They may laugh with me, but they always have my back. Even the dermatologist, amused as he may have been by my error, still wiped the ink from my nose before letting me walk back into the world. That's good medicine, and I take comfort in it.

17

Don't Burst My Bubble

Sometime over that first COVID summer, when the months of pandemic restrictions had stretched my creativity thin, I decided that I *had* to make giant bubbles. My mother had given my children a bubble kit a few years back, and I remembered enjoying it so much at the time that I wanted to try to recreate the magic. The only snag was that most recipes for giant bubbles required glycerin, which I didn't have on hand.

Glycerin is a fascinating substance. I know of no other compound that can be used in such varied things as bombs, baked goods, and bubbles. It's the Renaissance man of the chemical world. Since the grocery store didn't carry it and our local explosives supplier had been shuttered by the coronavirus, I tried my luck at the drugstore.

"Check in the laxative aisle," the clerk told me when I asked where I might find it. At the time I had been unaware of glycerin's use as a stool softener, so I found the suggestion a touch ridiculous, but sure enough, there it was in the laxative aisle, next to the castor oil and the Dulcolax.

My options were limited to a tub of solid glycerin suppositories or a four-pack of liquid ones. I briefly considered buying the giant tub and melting the contents down, but I wasn't sure if this was even possible, and I feared that having "Can I melt down glycerin suppositories" in my internet search history might put me on some kind of government watch list. Plus, I wasn't quite sure how I'd explain to my family what I was doing. I imagined myself standing over our sauce pot saying something like, "These would normally go in your butt, kids, but I'm cooking them down for bubbles. Also, who wants spaghetti for dinner?"

I opted for the liquid suppositories instead. Since I didn't know how much glycerin I needed for the project, I bought four packs—16 doses total—just to be safe. In retrospect, this was a lot of suppositories. I'm surprised the clerk didn't immediately pull me aside and call a doctor on my behalf.

Seeing all of the laxatives laid out on the conveyor belt reminded me of a time, years ago, when I had sent my husband out for an oral laxative to treat our toddler's constipation, only to have him return with an enema instead.

"I wanted the drink," I said, shaking my head. "I won't be able to do this."

"It's ok," my husband said. "I told him that you were going to give him a butt tickler."

I stared at him.

"You said *what*?"

"Like at the allergist?" he said, slowly backing away from me as his words finally settled into his ears.

It was true that a few months prior I had told our son that the allergist was going to "tickle his back" with some small needles for a skin prick test, and he laughed through the entire procedure. I had considered it a ringing endorsement for the power of suggestion, so I understood my husband's logic. "Butt tickling," however, just didn't translate. But everything worked out in the end, so to speak.

For a moment, I considered telling this story to the clerk (because who doesn't love hearing a good constipation story from a stranger?), but I decided to keep it to myself. Friends who know me might find the anecdote entertaining. A stranger might call the authorities. Still, the memory amused me.

I have since discovered that glycerin is available inexpensively and in non-suppository form at any craft store. Live and learn. When all was said and done, however, the drugstore glycerin worked just fine, and my daughter and I took turns making bubbles while the boys made a game of popping them with a Frisbee. Even the dog joined in. It was just the kind of simple fun I had hoped for. You might even say it tickled me. Though where, exactly, is none of your business.

18

A Christmas Miracle

My daughter and I attended a holiday party over the week-end, and as she and her friends worked on decorating ginger-bread houses, I was doing my level best to have a normal conversation with the other moms. I only knew one person at the party, and I was hoping to shield the others from my quirkiness, at least for an hour or two.

At one point, one of the women was admiring the host's Christmas tree and expressed her disappointment that she couldn't have a real tree at home because her husband is allergic to them.

"How does he manage to survive living in Washington?" I asked, genuinely curious, since there's no shortage of ever-green trees in this neck of the woods.

"Oh, poor guy, he's miserable all of the time!"

"I'm miserable all of the time, too, but I don't have such a handy excuse," I said.

No one in the room knew me well enough for that com-ment to spark concern, so everyone laughed. For a half beat I considered saying—in the deadpan way I've mastered over the years—"Why are you all laughing?" But I kept my mouth shut.

My goal for the afternoon was to keep things from getting awkward. The deadpan joke would have moved me from the mildly-depressed-and-funny category to mildly-depressed-and-weird. It's a minor miracle that I recognized this in the moment rather than just as the words were escaping my mouth, which, historically, has always been when I become painfully aware of my gaffes.

In almost every social situation, most of my internal monologue involves me repeating "Don't say it, don't say it. Oh, good Lord, don't say it" until I ignore the voice and say the thing anyway. The only time I can recall *not* saying anything when I was tempted to was when I was out shopping for houseplants and an old woman caught me eyeing a Dracaena that was on sale.

"They call that 'mother-in-law's tongue'," she said with a smirk, pausing before delivering her punchline. "Because it's so sharp."

In the space between her punchline and my response, my internal voice said flatly, "My mother-in-law is dead."

I desperately wanted to deliver this line aloud, but the woman was so pleased with herself and her joke that I couldn't bear the thought of skewering her in this way. Plus, I could clearly see my future self in her, spending my days stalking unsuspecting customers at the plant nursery, waiting to spring my best horticultural jokes on them. So I simply laughed politely and said, "Is that right?" It was a small victory for normalcy.

I'm constantly struggling against my instincts in my efforts to appear normal. I was once telling friends a story of some embarrassing situation I had gotten myself into, and as I was lamenting the fact that I had failed so miserably at being my best self in that situation, I accidentally said "my breast self." We had such a good laugh over this that I adopted the phrase as part of a personal credo of sorts: "Be your best self, not your breast self," I often say, which is my way of encouraging myself not to be a boob.

I'm not always successful. One of my favorite baristas at the local coffee roaster I frequent is a young "lumbersexual" man who sports a bushy beard on what otherwise appears to be a baby face. Because of this incongruity, I had absolutely no idea how old he might be. One day, against my better judgment (as always) I decided to ask him. It went something like this:

"How old are you, if you don't mind me asking?" (Looking back, this would have been a good stopping point) "Because you look so young, but I can't tell with your beard and all."

At that moment, after discovering I could have been this kid's mother, my question suddenly felt vaguely inappropriate, like I'd wondered aloud if a beard like that would scratch or tickle. I babbled on nervously for a bit.

"It's getting so hard to tell ages anymore, since you boys are wearing all that facial hair." I grabbed my latte and hightailed it out of the place before I could say anything else.

Later, after telling the story to my husband, he teased me mercilessly about the interaction.

"Did Mama want a mustache ride?"

"Don't be a creep," I said, swatting him with a dish towel. "He only had a beard."

Most days, I spend a good bit of time apologizing to people I've talked to in social settings and mentally rehearsing how to interact with acquaintances I might run into in the cheese aisle of the grocery store. It turns out that having had nothing but parasocial relationships with television characters in my formative years might have stunted my social development a bit. But if the Christmas party is any indication, I'm making a bit of progress in the awkwardness department. I'm learning to apply my editing skills to conversation. *Less is more* has been the biggest takeaway from my many odd encounters. I still expect to be my breast self on occasion, but I think I've succeeded in bringing myself down a cup size or two.

I had hoped that by middle age I would have shed the remains of my adolescent self-consciousness in favor of a more mature self-confidence. I have always longed to know what it feels like to walk into a room and *own* it, to have an internal voice that says things like *Everyone here is looking at me because I'm someone who commands attention* instead of *Everyone here is looking at me because I have toilet paper tucked into my pantyhose, don't I?*

I don't know that I'll ever learn to fully quiet that self-conscious voice, but as I get older, I'm trying to be more mindful of how much space I give it. And I'm learning to adjust my expectations for social interactions so that I can stop viewing myself as the socially inept one by default. I know that I am under no obligation to be pleasing or entertaining or even safely, blandly ordinary for anyone. That knowledge doesn't seem to stop me from wanting to be all of those things, however.

Once I am able to fully absorb that lesson, to let go of my concerns about other people's perceptions of me, I think I'll finally *feel* less awkward, even if I remain as awkward as I've ever been. Maybe then I will be able to retrain that internal voice of mine to say not *They're laughing at you because you're an ass* but *They're laughing because you are a delightful person who is as real as they come.* In the end, being real is what matters. A carefully crafted image might get you followers. Authenticity, however, will get you genuine friends.

19

Thou Shalt Not Covet Thy Neighbor's Cat

A few winters ago, I was actively engaged in a plot to steal my neighbor's cat. I can't say that cat theft was in my plans when I sat down to think about my resolutions for the year, but these kinds of temptations tend to rise up of their own accord.

It all began innocently enough. One morning, I discovered a pretty little gray and white cat sitting at my front door crying to get in. It was an uncharacteristically cold winter, and, fearing he might be a stray, I let him in and fed him some smoked salmon that I happened to have in the fridge. That was all it took for the daily visits to begin.

He was a sweet cat. Every day, he'd come by and let me snuggle him for a few minutes before perching himself on the back of the couch where he could watch the birds peck at the shrubs outside of the front window. After a few hours, he'd sit at the door and cry to be let out, so I would oblige him and then go on about my day. He was pleasant company at a time when I desperately needed it, and I began to think that I was meant to keep him, as if the universe had sent this cat to me to help ease my loneliness. He didn't even trigger my son's allergies, which only served to fortify my belief that my relationship with this cat was, indeed, kismet.

I made a feeble attempt to see if this cat had an owner, but even this half-hearted effort easily revealed that he belonged to a woman down the street. She told me her cat's name was Gray Kitty, though the neighborhood children had taken to calling him Frank, and he had been unhappy since she added a dog to the household over the summer. She asked me to stop letting him in so that he wouldn't get too settled with me and I agreed, but when he showed up each morning, I would think to myself, *He's clearly trying to move out of his house*, and I'd let him in anyway. The heart wants what it wants. Who was I to stand in the way?

Before long, I bought a litter box and a bag of cat food—*You know, just in case I can't get him to go home some night*—I explained to my husband, who didn't even register a note of disapproval with this plan as he sat on the couch taking selfies with said cat. It was a good choice, as he did stay over a night or two, burrowing under my covers to sleep curled up next to my feet. I had never been much of a cat person, but Gray Kitty had me completely smitten.

I must have reeked of desperation though, because just as quickly as my smoked salmon had lured him into my life, the litter box sent him running for the hills. That level of commitment proved to be too much too soon, and he disappeared as fast as a man spooked by the discovery of his girlfriend's toothbrush in his apartment. Gray Kitty would still come around the house occasionally, but he'd never come in. He'd just stare at me with a look that said something like *I thought we were keeping things casual.*

He showed up on my doorstep a few weeks ago, obviously unaware that I had moved on and invited a dog to live with me. When Chino spotted him through the glass, he stopped dead and stared with a look of indignant disbelief. It took him a few beats to collect himself enough to begin barking, which succeeded in chasing away the intruder. But before Gray Kitty turned to run off, likely for the last time, I could swear I detected just a hint of regret in his eyes, and it pleased me.

20

Cowboy Songs

As I sat down to lunch yesterday, I found myself singing an old cowboy tune, "I've Got Spurs That Jingle Jangle Jingle." I can't claim to be a big fan of the Western genre, but for reasons that remain a mystery to me, I had to learn this song in an elementary school music class. It's an odd choice for children. The lyrics tell the story of a man who is constantly shrugging off women who'd like to ensnare him in domestic life, and in the chorus, he gently croons to each heartbroken girl that he can't settle down because life on the range is the only life for him:

> *I've got spurs that jingle, jangle, jingle*
> *As I go riding merrily along*
> *And they sing, oh, ain't you glad you're single?*
> *And that song ain't so very far from wrong.*

It's a cheery little tune, and I must have enjoyed singing it as a child, considering I still sing it to myself on occasion as an adult. Still, I can't even imagine what the teacher might have told us about the lyrics. Did she use the singer as an exemplar of some sort, a model for the boys to follow? Did she warn us girls to avoid trying to trap men in general or cowboys specifically? I can't recall. Maybe she just let out a world-weary sigh and said, "Ack. Men," then shook her head and dismissed us from class.

That same year we also learned the song "Whoopee Ti-Yi-Yo, Git Along Little Dogies," which is about a cattle drive from Texas to Wyoming. Mind you, I grew up in Pennsylvania, which is not exactly a hotbed of cattle ranching (though we did have a neighbor who raised cow-bison hybrids we called "beefalo"). This song is so deeply embedded in my brain that I sang it incessantly the moment my family crossed the border into Wyoming during a road trip a few summers ago, much to everyone's chagrin. I had expected my husband to be able to sing along with me, but I was surprised to learn that he did not also possess my extensive knowledge of cowboy ballads.

Despite having grown up in Colorado, where there are *actual cowboys* tending to proper cattle ranches rather than 4H kids raising a few beefalo to sell at the county fair, my husband couldn't so much as *ti yi yippee yippee yay* with me. I was perplexed.

"It's from 'The Old Chisholm Trail,'" I said. "You didn't learn this in elementary school?"

He shook his head.

"What about 'Texas Ranger'? 'Blood on the Saddle'? Anything?"

Crickets.

I couldn't believe this was not common knowledge to us

both. I had always assumed Western music was one of those odd little pieces of Americana that children were required to learn in primary school in the 1980s—much like square dancing. But it turns out that a good chunk of my early musical education was shaped by one middle-aged teacher's obsession with cowboys.

Though my husband and I didn't learn the same American folk tunes in school, we both inexplicably learned the Australian bush ballad "Waltzing Matilda." In it, a transient man steals a sheep to eat for dinner, then, when confronted by the law, elects to drown himself in the billabong rather than be hauled off to jail. His ghost then haunts the watering hole for all eternity. In short, it has all of the elements of a great story for eight-year-olds.

We puzzled over the reasons that children from Pennsylvania to Colorado would have learned this song in school. It might have ticked the box for a 1980s version of cultural diversity—Australia was foreign but still comfortably English speaking and white (save for their aboriginal people who, like our own, were largely invisible at the time). Plus, we could use words like billabong and jumbuck and think ourselves worldly without going through the trouble of actually traveling the world or learning a new language. It was public school's answer to the problems of class.

The most logical explanation, we finally concluded, was that a small cohort of younger Gen X kids was being brainwashed to be government operatives, and "Waltzing Matilda" was chosen as our post-hypnotic trigger. One day the tune would be played over the radio, layered under one of the emergency broadcast tests, and all of us who were raised on movies like *Red Dawn* and *War Games* (which, in retrospect, look remarkably like training guides for child assassins) would pick up our weapons and take down some Commies before heading home for dinner, blissfully unaware of what we'd done in "school" that day. I've read stranger conspiracy theories online.

In reality, we were probably singing these songs because they were fun. The jingle jangling of the cowboy's spurs taught us the concept of onomatopoeia and that was that. We had neither the language nor experience to think of the singer as a cad for how he treated his poor lady friends; we could just feel the freedom of those wide-open spaces that he cherished. We learned the songs because they had upbeat melodies or because the teacher liked them or because—in the case of "Waltzing Matilda"—they were filled with silly sounding words that were English. . .but not quite. What a fun idea to explore as a child, that life is filled with nuance of all kinds—like discovering that your crayfish are your Southern cousin's crawdads, or that your beloved Edy's ice cream is Dreyer's west of the Rockies. We may each see the world from a slant, but the world itself remains wondrous and joyful.

A few years ago, my family took a trip to a Texas dude ranch in order to escape the gloom of the Pacific Northwest in February. We rode horses to breakfast each morning, where the "cowboys" would cook for us over an open fire, and one of the camp hands serenaded us with his guitar as we ate. I recognized one of his tunes from my childhood and sang along under my breath. Though I knew the dude ranch was meant to be a sort of simulacrum of the frontier experience, in that moment, singing along to that familiar old tune, I felt a genuine connection to the history of the place. It may have taken 30 years or so, but those elementary school lessons had finally paid off.

Before the performer finished his song, he caught me singing along and offered me a friendly wink. I smiled back and thought of my old music teacher.

No use trying to lasso this one, Miss Ianucci, I thought. Though she sure might have had some fun trying.

21

Oh Captain, My Captain

"You can be my captain any day," the old man said to me, rifle in hand, his VFW side cap perched at a precarious angle over a wild tuft of hair, all of it hopelessly out of regulation. As the officer in charge of the military funeral we were prepping for, I briefly considered telling him to drop for a few pushups as a teasing way to reprimand him for getting fresh, but his big doe eyes were so imploring that I feared he might actually do it just to impress me, and the exertion might very well have killed him, ancient as he was. I wasn't in the mood to oversee two funerals that day.

Instead, I settled for a response that was more playful than lethal.

"Today's your lucky day then," I said with a wink, partly to give him the little thrill he was after and partly to inspire him to put himself together for the ceremony. The wink was a gamble. It wasn't quite conduct unbefitting of an officer, but it may have been a bit unseemly, considering I was about to preside over a funeral, though the deceased was a

WWII veteran who had been the volunteer rifleman's friend and would likely have approved of his old buddy's flirtation, especially since he succeeded in getting this wink out of me. Decorum doesn't seem to concern men too much as they get older. The fight-to-the-death impulse of their youth gradually morphs into flirt-to-the-death, even if it means flirting at your best friend's funeral. What better place to remind a man that time is of the essence.

I've noticed that some men become relentlessly flirtatious as they get older, and truth be told, I love this about them. Since there's nothing in the way of romance at stake, it's possible to simply enjoy the spirit of these exchanges. If I'm being perfectly honest, I still enjoy the attention, even if I know that these men will lavish it on any woman within earshot who is willing to listen to them speak. I love the unhurried, easy cadence to an old man's stories and the over-the-top compliments offered up solely to elicit a smile. Sentimental fool that I am, I find them charming.

My receptivity to these advances must somehow be obvious, because old men chat me up wherever I go. I'd like to attribute this to some mysterious allure of mine, the side effect of being a Scorpio perhaps, but I imagine it has more to do with the fact that I am middle-aged than anything else. I am of Safe Flirting Age—that is, not too young to invite much tongue clucking from anyone who might see us chatting.

It might also have something to do with the fact that I'll often engage in a little banter with strange men, even when I'm obviously being catcalled rather than complimented. Such was the case in my local public library, when a man I passed by on the stairs made a few appreciative sounds, the kind most people reserve for food, and said, "Your husband must be so proud." I looked him directly in the eye and said, "He's satisfied, too." Then I winked and disappeared into the stacks, ever the woman of mystery.

In any event, I think it's mostly my friendly face that attracts attention. While I was waiting on my order at a coffee shop one morning, an older gentleman approached and advised me to avoid breaking my wrist, nodding toward the brace on his hand as proof that he was an expert on such matters. It was conversational bait I'd never heard before, and even though the poor-injured-man bit was one of Ted Bundy's favorite ploys and should have set off some alarm bells, I took it.

"I'll try my best," I said, at which point the man went into great detail about how he had injured himself in a mountain biking accident the week before. He showed me some of the scars he had collected over the years, noting that they were the reason he had to settle for doing "stupid safe shit" in his old age.

"Like mountain biking?" I asked, sincerely puzzled, since it's high on my mental list of activities that might land my teenage son in the emergency room. But maybe it gets safer as the frontal lobe develops. He couldn't tell me either way.

There was an undercurrent of loss to this man's story that resonated with me. I knew that in telling it he was simply asking me to see him, to picture more than just a battle-scarred old man in a coffee shop. He was asking me see the entirety of his life, to imagine who he was in his more daring and virile youth. I'm familiar enough with this feeling that I was happy to oblige him.

When he was through lamenting the fact that he'd soon have to worry about breaking a hip rather than a wrist, he sighed and said, "You've probably broken a few bones during this journey of life, so you know how it is." He put his hand on my shoulder. "As beautiful as you are, I'm sure you've broken a few hearts at least."

This was the most elaborate set-up for a line I'd ever heard, and I was impressed. I tilted my head and smiled.

"Oh, you," I said, swatting him on his uninjured arm.

It was all like some ritual performed by instinct, the scripts to these exchanges written into our genes. We are merely asked to play our respective roles on occasion, easing each other's longing to be seen. There's a certain intimacy to this kind of connection, and I always feel more at one with humanity as a whole whenever I experience it. When I put it this way to my husband, he gently suggested I stop connecting so deeply with these men.

I won't though. I've always been fond of old men, possibly because I was very close to my grandfather and am now drawn to the same kind of impish energy he possessed. I love to observe them, to see how the relief from all the burdens of their youth has helped them ease into their skin over time. There's so little self-consciousness to an old man. There's no other way to explain their wild eyebrows and workout jeans. I long to be so self-assured.

It may be this sense of ease that intrigues me about these men—and women, too, frankly. Whereas men become more flirtatious as they age, women seem to become more irreverent, and I love that quality equally. I admire the way these elder men and women have succeeded in drawing the world's attention inward at a time when it no longer fixes its gaze on their physical form. It can be tempting to simply mourn the loss of our youth and vigor and retreat from the world as we age rather than honor the humor, kindness, passion, and intelligence we carry within us, the qualities that have always been the true measures of our worth, whether or not anyone recognized them.

I try to look inward as much as I can, to peek behind the veil of these facades we construct for ourselves—and that sometimes are constructed *for* us—so that I might truly see people. It's not enough to only be seen, after all; we need to be understood. During that funeral detail years ago, I had the sense that the man who was so eager to call me captain wanted my approval more than anything else. I kept that in mind as the day wore on.

At the conclusion of the funeral service, the honor guard fired their volleys, three shots to signal that the dead had been cleared from the battle field and would be cared for. The riflemen weren't perfectly in sync—years spent in the artillery and simple old age had deteriorated their hearing—but they were square-jawed and solemn, hard men still. Bits of their younger selves had been dusted off for the occasion, which was obvious enough to anyone who might have taken a moment to notice.

After the ceremony, I shook hands with the men and congratulated them on a job well done. I could almost see a hint of the boy my doe-eyed friend had once been as he took my hand and beamed.

22

Past Lives of Our Parents

I was telling a well-worn story about my time in Germany when I mentioned in passing that I had lived there for three years.

"Three *years?*" my son said in mild disbelief. "I always thought you were there on vacation."

I laughed at this, not only because his reaction revealed an almost stunning lack of awareness of what my life was like before children but because he had used this exact tone and phrasing to interject into a conversation I was having with his sister about puberty. He overheard me say that menstruation lasts, on average, three to five days (or up to ten if you're trying to avoid your husband's advances).

"Five *days?*" he said, in that same incredulous tone. "I thought it lasted, like, an hour."

I can't fault my son for not being able to relate to me as someone other than Mom, nor do I fault him for being some-what oblivious to the particulars of the menstrual cycle—he has no reason to care about either thing at the moment. That will come in due time.

Nevertheless, if I'm being perfectly honest, I was a bit hurt that he didn't know more about me. I've done some interesting things through the years, and I had hoped that a few of my stories might have captured his imagination. But adolescence is an egocentric stage of life, I realize, and I guess it's better that he's more focused on his abs at the moment than on how to understand his mother.

The kids might know more about me if I weren't raising them 3,000 miles away from where I grew up and an ocean away from where I spent the bulk of my time in the Army. From this distance, there's simply no one around to offer them a glimpse into my pre-domestic life. There are no Sunday dinners with Grandma where she regales them with tales of my girlhood antics, no old flames passing by us on the street. Sometimes I wish we lived in one of my former haunts solely so that I might one day run into an ex and introduce him to my children—in a voice that in my head sounds like a faintly British Katherine Hepburn—as "Mummy's former *lover*." Then I'd laugh and laugh as they all melted into a puddle of humiliation beside me.

But even without any of this external prompting, every now and then we'll get a glimpse of our parents as the people they were before they had children, and it can be a bit jarring to realize that they had—and continue to have—identities other than Mom and Dad. Biology must somehow ensure that we avoid thinking of our forebears this way. My husband recalls a time during his childhood when he was shocked to learn that his father—a bit soft around the middle and seemingly less-than-athletic at the time—had once been a star baseball player and a college football recruit before an injury curtailed his college sports career.

For me, it was my grandmother who forced this reckoning. I had always thought of her as an old-fashioned woman, particularly with regard to sex and sexuality. She had adopted the prudish mother persona that was expected of women in the 50s and 60s, her three children arriving only because she had the fortitude to grit her teeth and bear the indignities of her wifely duties, not because she'd enjoyed even a moment of their conception. So when, in my early 20s, I finally heard her make a direct reference to sex, specifically to the power it allowed women to wield over men, I was momentarily taken aback. *You mean to tell me that Grandma was a* woman *before she was my grandmother?* It was a revelation.

The very idea that my husband's father once possessed some athletic prowess had been as unimaginable to him as the image of my grandmother as some *femme fatale* had been to me. To acknowledge that they once had these qualities was to also accept that they eventually lost them. Perhaps this is really why we're reluctant to investigate our parents' early lives too deeply. We'd prefer to hold fast to the illusion of our own eternal youth and invincibility.

But I'll *always be active and fit and cool enough to hang with the younger crowd* we insist to ourselves as we embark on our parenting journeys, ignoring all evidence that prior generations have provided to the contrary. Then one morning we wake up and find that we have managed to injure ourselves while sleeping and the children begin to shrink away from us when their friends are around and we're beginning to notice our parents' gestures and phrases escaping our own bodies against our will. Maybe this new common ground is enough to make us wonder if our parents had, in fact, once been like us after all, misspending their youth in the same unfortunate ways. Only then can we finally understand each other, and the parenting process is complete.

~

A few years ago, my son told me that he wasn't looking forward to returning to school because the girls would always chase him on the playground.

"You just don't know what that's like, Mom," he said, happily unaware of the fact that anyone might have chased his mother in years past. Some day he will come to understand that I was a woman as well as his mother, with dreams and desires that were sometimes at odds with the role I assumed when he was born.

But on that day, I was just Mom—safe haven and healer of wounds both physical and emotional, a steady presence in a confusing world. Even if he should never see me as anything other than these things, it seems my life will have been well spent playing this part. In that moment, listening to him worry aloud about the girls at school, I saw no reason to shatter his illusion that his mother was all I might be.

"You're right, Son," I said, patting his hand and offering a sympathetic look as I recalled my own younger days of chasing and being chased. "That must be very frustrating."

23

Always Carry a Hankie

I wound up crying in Jimmy John's today. It wasn't the 1000 calories of grease I was shoving into my face or the fact that I was supporting big game hunting with my purchase that led to my crying jag; rather, it was a sign on the wall that got me. It read, "The happiest people don't *have* the best of everything, they *make* the best of everything." It was one of those trite sayings that would typically make me roll my eyes, but for some reason, today, it struck a sentimental chord. I felt embarrassed enough about this to laugh a bit before the tears came on in full force, and I tried at first to disguise my crying as laughter. In the end, I couldn't find anything funny enough nearby to blame for laughing to the point of tears, so I eventually just confessed to my family that I was crying about the sign.

My husband looked at the sign, then at me, bemused.

"What evolutionary purpose could this possibly serve?" he wondered aloud.

I've given him plenty of reasons to question this. Though

I've always been easily moved to tears, over the last few months the waterworks have been more unpredictable and freely flowing than usual. I am not pregnant, so I can only assume this has been due to normal age-related hormone changes, thus my husband's musing.

Not long ago, while watching *The Biggest Little Farm*, I found myself overwhelmed when one of the farmers plunged her hands into living soil where there had once been only hardpan. I was alone in the theater and didn't have anyone to share this wave of emotion with, so I just sat there in the dark, straight-up sobbing while I muttered "It's so beautiful" to myself. A few weeks later, I had a particularly powerful reaction to the Dave's Killer Bread story, which I was reading aloud from the side of the bread bag. I was touched to learn how the company supports ex-convicts through second-chance employment.

"It's just so nice," I began, already choking on my words, which prompted a sideways glance from Chad. "Without a community (sniff) the recidivism rate (sniff) is so (sniff) hi-hi-hi-hiiiiiiiiigh." Then I proceeded to cry on my toast.

Though the biological link between hormones and mood is relatively clear, I have also considered Chad's question about the purpose of mood swings during this phase of life. He offered up a hypothesis that in the "grandma" years (biologically speaking), women could use an extra dose of empathy and compassion to support their grandchildren and therefore tend to have heightened responses to the smallest emotional triggers. When I posed this question to friends, one woman suggested the mood swings were designed to send our partners off to "younger and more fertile soils." I laughed at this. Until I cried.

In the end, I doubt there is an evolutionary benefit at all. Not all women suffer from mood swings in the years leading up to menopause, and for those who do, it is one of those unfortunate traits that only reveals itself after the childbearing years have all but ended, ensuring that the weepiness genes will survive into the next generation.

Maybe I didn't inherit the best of genes in this department. That's fine. Like my good friend Jimmy John always says whenever he bags a leopard instead of a lion, you just have to make the best of things. I can at least laugh my way through this season of life. Sometimes the laughter might even help to disguise the tears.

24

On the Burdens of Sex

Off the top of my head, I can think of a handful of men in their sixties and beyond who are managing to hold fast to their sex appeal. My own father issues notwithstanding, these men are objectively handsome. They are rugged, accomplished, and fit, and their wrinkles communicate both a sense of gravitas and financial security. The allure of a hefty 401k is undeniable.

I've been drawn to older men ever since I was a child, when I had an inexplicable crush on Telly Savalas of *Kojak* fame. Admitting to this was a small consolation to my husband, who could take it as proof that I'm not lying about my fondness for bald men, but it was of no consolation to me. In fact, the more I think about my attraction to older men, the more infuriated I get by it. It's the lack of reciprocity that burns me up. Should I reach my sixties, there certainly won't be any men in their forties looking at me with anything resembling lust. They won't be looking at me at all, since women just fade away after menopause as if they're gradually being erased from existence by some foolhardy time traveler. Meanwhile, my husband can look forward to being desired by women young and old for all time.

I'm hardly the jealous type, but I can't stomach the thought of competing for him twenty years from now, after a long marriage and all of its attendant familiarities. I might be able to hold my own against women my age, but I simply won't be able to compete with anyone younger. How could I? Who wants a prune when a plum is right there, practically bursting with juice? The prune always loses unless the prune is a man. Sometimes I'll look at the wrinkles around my husband's eyes, think them oddly attractive, and just seethe.

Whenever I begin carping about the injustice of men's eternal sex appeal though, my husband can barely keep from rolling his seductive wrinkled eyes at me.

"You're forgetting how easy it is for women to have sex overall," he said. "From 18 to 30, all you have to do is say the word. Men always have to work for it when they're young."

I might have winced a bit at the age bracket he rattled off so casually, as if a dozen odd years ago he finally breathed a sigh of relief knowing he didn't have to worry about other men sniffing around his dried-up 30-year-old wife, but I saw his point. Before I could even open my mouth to concede, he continued on his rant.

"Plus, when we're older, younger women only want us because we have money."

"So you're saying you'd only enjoy having sex with younger women if they wanted *you* and not your money?"

He paused for a second to think. "Of course not," he laughed. "I'm just saying that men don't become more physically desirable as they get older. You're thinking about this the wrong way."

"They just acquire more desirable traits," I finished, nodding. "Fair enough."

~

On some ancient genetic level, we're likely programmed to behave in this way. Women recognize that older men offer security and stability. They're a safe bet to have children with, as they're less likely than younger men to go out for cigarettes and wander off for good. When my second great-grandmother became an unwed teenage mother at the turn of the twentieth century, her parents married her off to a neighbor man nearly thirty years her senior precisely because of the stability (and more children) he could provide for her. That's all understandable. But the very fact that men can father children until they die seems to be one of the most profoundly unfair differences between the sexes.

Former President John Tyler, born in 1790, still had a *grandson* walking this earth in 2020 thanks to this biological advantage of men. Tyler fathered his last child at 63, and that child was still fathering children into his *mid-seventies*, creating a generation gap wide as the Sargasso Sea. My own grandfather fathered his last child at age 64, so this is not the exclusive domain of wealthy and powerful men. Remaining sexually relevant into old age is an achievable dream for any average Joe, making it all the more maddening.

More than men's enduring desirability, it's this utility piece that bothers me. As women, we are given a biological expiration date, after which point we effectively become useless to the species. Even when science intervenes to upend this limitation, as it did for a 74-year-old Indian woman who gave birth to twins via IVF in 2019, moral outrage tends to ensue. Critics of geriatric pregnancies claim that women are incapable of caring for a baby at an advanced age, but they have no similar concerns about elderly fathers. Geriatric fatherhood is part of the natural order of things. At best, older women can care for grandchildren whose young fathers never return from their cigarette run, but they can't continue adding to the gene pool as men can. But in that regard, given the investment of time and energy we have to make to carry, birth, and raise a child, we've always had to privilege quality over quantity. Without at least one party acting discerningly, men would just be sowing their seed everywhere, without the slightest thought to the kind of the fruit they're producing. I guess women's role as quality control is vital enough, though decidedly less fun.

Neither gender is inherently privileged over the other, at least as far as nature is concerned. We each have our burdens to bear, and my husband was right to find my complaint about older men's desirability annoying. As a young woman holding all of the sexual power, I had never, not once, thought about the insecurity that young men must feel on occasion about their own attractiveness and worth, since the role of pursuer naturally comes with ample rejection. I had only begun to consider this particular dynamic when I felt that power shifting out of my hands. I'm a bit embarrassed to admit that I had never considered my husband's point because I had been too busy wallowing in self-pity over my own aging process.

This supposed injustice of an older man's sex appeal is not really an injustice at all. It's only fair that the pendulum should swing in this direction, given all the years young men have to suffer the pain of their unfulfilled needs, left alone with only their yearning and their lotion. Nature has a way of maintaining equilibrium, whether or not we choose to recognize it as such.

It's of little comfort to know that old men are simply having their day when our day has already come and gone. Aging for women can be brutal. I was once watching an improv show that Florence Henderson was making a guest appearance on. She looked great for her age, but she had lost the youthful dewiness she'd had when she was starring in *The Brady Bunch*. She'd dulled to more of a matte finish, but I've always found a certain elegance to that look.

The moderator had set up some kind of sexually suggestive scene between Ms. Henderson and one of the younger actors, and immediately, as if by instinct, the young man cringed at the thought. Cringed! To his credit, he recognized his gaffe and appeared sheepish about it, but the truth had already been written all over his face: the very idea of sleeping with an older woman disgusted him. Had the roles been reversed, it's entirely possible that a young female actor would have leaned into the sexual nature of the scene, might have asked the old man to spank her for being a naughty girl. Everyone would have laughed, and it all would have been good fun. Not so for poor Carol Brady.

I was about to try arguing that this actor's response in the skit was just more evidence that older women are unfairly judged by the opposite sex, but then I thought back to my own younger days yet again. How many times had I deemed a man unworthy—not tall enough or strong enough, not even a tuft of chest hair to prove he's got enough testosterone in his bloodstream? I had been making the same assessments that this actor had, though more politely.

Still, I never want to feel that my body is repulsive, even if I do accept that my desirability will fade over time. Perhaps this is the upside of finding older men attractive: I always get to be the younger woman with them. Should my husband ever heed the call of his hormones and take off for more fertile ground, I can at least take comfort in knowing I could always find an older husband. The arrangement doesn't seem half bad at that, a little twist on the traditional set-up I've enjoyed for most of my adult life: I'd have one last chance to feel young and beautiful again, while simultaneously having a place to channel my motherly instincts—lying fallow after the children have grown and gone—into caring for my new, aging spouse. Then, when my husband departs for the next world, leaving me with his retirement fund to do with as I please, Chad will be changing diapers with his new young bride while I am sleeping in each morning, with only my stolen cats to tend to. Just as nature intended.

25

Shifting the Gaze

I was walking my dog around a local college campus when I heard a rowdy group of students running through the woods. As they approached, I noticed that the young men leading the pack appeared to be completely naked. It was close to fraternity rush time, so I assumed I was witnessing some kind of hazing ritual, a pledge class being forced to streak across the campus perhaps, but I wasn't fully prepared to encounter nudity on my afternoon walk, and I froze. Once the group fully emerged from the bushes, however, it was clear—to my relief—that they were wearing Speedos.

Don't interpret my relief to mean I'm a prude. I'm far from it. There's nothing about the human body that I object to seeing, but as this throng of half-clothed boys descended upon me in the woods, I couldn't help but realize how *young* they all were and how fixing my gaze on them would be uncomfortable for all of us and borderline criminal for me. So I just stood there, awkwardly staring at the dog, who had plopped himself down in the grass in total confusion, until the runners passed by.

Had they been slightly older men, or even a mix of these man-children and older men, I probably would have helped myself to a better look had they been running in the buff, not because I'd have found it titillating necessarily, but I'd at least have been interested to note how circumcision trends have changed through the years. More than that, I would have wanted to satisfy my curiosity about how men run with their particular anatomy in the first place. Given the production my son makes about the slightest hit to the crotch, I have trouble understanding how such a high-impact sport doesn't mercilessly abuse the gonads.

I was averting my gaze but still thinking an awful lot about testicles and such, probably more than any middle-aged woman who is not a urologist should. They mystify me to be honest, despite having spent 20-odd years getting acquainted with them. I imagine the reverse is also true for men, who might be able to draw a rough sketch of the Mound of Venus and its environs but can never fully appreciate what it's like to actually be in possession of a vagina. We are utterly unknowable to one another.

It's natural to be curious about anything that is foreign to us, even more so if that thing happens to be somewhat taboo. We need only think back to childhood to find examples, when bodies were an endless source of fascination. Whenever my cousins would visit as I was growing up, we'd casually pull down one particular volume of the *Life Cycle Library* from my bookshelf and steal away with it. Then, huddled together in some secluded corner of the house, we'd find the page with the full-frontal illustration of a naked boy and immediately fall apart laughing. My aunt broke into our huddle one day to see what could possibly be entertaining us so much. She peered over our shoulders then looked at Frankie—the only boy among us—and flatly asked him if he laughed at himself whenever he went to the bathroom.

How could you not laugh? I wonder now. Every time my family goes backpacking and my husband and son get to pee freely in the wilderness, I think: How could you not laugh with glee at the sheer ease of everything that comes with having a penis? It's truly a marvel.

But that's a different issue. Besides, we were laughing derisively back then, even Frankie was. What did he find laughable about this depiction of himself? We were mainly laughing because we were engaged in a low-level scandal by looking at a naked body, true, but we were also laughing at the body itself. There's something, well, just *funny* about the male anatomy. I have even heard grown men, *professional men*, men who are otherwise exemplars of decorum and class, make the occasional penis joke. When compared to the soft, mysterious bodies of their female counterparts, I suppose all of the exposed dangly bits make obvious subjects for commentary. Plus, the equipment seems slightly confounding at times, even to its owners, so maybe it's therapeutic to laugh about it.

Still, there's a self-consciousness to this joking that pulls at my heartstrings a bit. I told my husband my concerns: In thinking about our tendency to make a joke of the male form,

I began to wonder if we've implicitly made a joke of men and masculinity in general.

"Do men feel more exposed and therefore more vulnerable in their intimate relationships because of this?" I asked.

Chad looked thoughtful before he responded.

"You know," he said, "until you mentioned it, I'd never really thought about what happens to it when I run."

He stared off into the distance, I assume to conjure the sensation of genitalia being jostled on a jog.

"I wear boxer briefs, so I guess it just finds its spot and stays there."

It seems I had been overthinking things, as usual. I closed my laptop, clearly finished with this topic for the time being. I smiled at my husband and patted him on the shoulder.

"Well, at least I finally have an answer to that question," I said.

26

On the Trail Again

One of the first things I learned about backpacking once my husband finally convinced me to go out on the trail was that four days spent subsisting on beans and beef jerky will test the constitution of any family, in every imaginable way. The children were twelve and nine when we first began venturing out in the wilderness for days at a time, as if beds and indoor plumbing were the stuff of fairy tales, but there was virtually no complaining about the miles of hiking or the heat or the bugs. Mostly we fought over which one of us would have to bring up the rear on the trail.

While I like being in the woods, I don't love backpacking. At best I can say that I enjoy *having backpacked*, in much the same way a woman might describe giving birth—it's mostly miserable but worth it in the end. In either case, you're left with bragging rights about how much pain you can endure.

I never feel more vulnerable, more at the world's mercy, than I do when we first set out on some remote mountain trail, cut off from the world while cougars stalk us from somewhere just out of sight. It's unnerving. The dangers we encounter on our trips pale in comparison to those found on the glaciated mountains though, where you might be happily trekking along and suddenly plunge into a crevasse, never to be seen again. But even on less treacherous terrain, I'm on edge almost the entire time we're outdoors.

My anxieties about being in the wilderness are new. I spent a good chunk of my childhood roaming the Pennsylvania woods like a feral animal, and I did so without a care. The woods were the rural equivalent of a play room, and adults would rarely bother me there. (It was the 1980s, so adults rarely bothered children anywhere.)

My father would often send me out on a mission to dig up mayapple roots or ginseng if I could find it, which he claimed to sell to some mysterious Asian root buyers he had connected with through an ad in the back of *Field and Stream*. Even back then the story seemed implausible, but as long as I got my cut of the proceeds, I didn't ask questions. I suspect he was just paying me to stay outside all day. As a parent, I appreciate the genius of this. Now my own children will venture off into the wild, happily schlepping twenty percent of their body weight without the slightest monetary incentive to do so. They are better children than I was, though less fiscally shrewd.

The Pennsylvania landscape seemed friendlier in my memory than the rugged terrain of the Pacific Northwest, even though we had mountain lions and bears and poisonous snakes back home as well. Maybe it seemed more inviting because I was just a dumb kid who was completely oblivious to the dangers that lurked in the shadows. I'm sure that now, as an anxious and world-wise adult, the Appalachian Trail would evoke the same feelings of smallness and vulnerability as the Pacific Crest Trail, since all of the dangers large and small have been exposed over time. But nature and I have formed a tentative alliance.

My children seem to feel none of this fear, none of the oppressive sense of insignificance that the wilderness tends to evoke in me. They are in their element outdoors, content to simply be, creating diversions from whatever nature offers them. Whenever the wild threatens to overwhelm me, I can, at the very least, appreciate my children's easy joy. I'd like to say that this alone makes the whole camping ordeal worthwhile, but I still have to dig a hole for a toilet in the backcountry, and I am only sentimental to a point.

I could wax poetic about all the things I do love about the outdoors, but sentiment tends to get lost in a fart cloud on the trail. Early on I warned my husband that if he wanted me to rough it in the wilderness, I'd give him a really close look at my animal nature, and I didn't mean that in a sexy way. It wouldn't be long before he'd come to appreciate the herculean effort it takes me at home to constantly shield him from some of my less attractive qualities. And that's without all of the dried beans. Unfortunately, this didn't dissuade him.

I was always taught that to preserve marital harmony and any hope for lasting desire, bodily functions must remain a mystery between partners. But backpacking upends that notion. It's impossible to sneak away from camp for your morning constitutional without everyone knowing what's up. *Yes, I've just had three cups of coffee, but I'm merely walking off to investigate an ant hill I saw yesterday. It will take me fifteen minutes to take adequate notes. Don't follow me because these ants can be quite dangerous.* At that point, the jig is up.

If you're looking to get closer to your family, there's no better place than the woods to do so. Backpacking has brought me so close to my husband that I now have an intimate knowledge of what okra does to his intestines, which I can say with some authority is more than any woman needs to know about her spouse. The same goes for the kids, whose high-altitude flatus emissions have woken them from a sound sleep, prompting a gagging argument over which one of them was responsible for the smell. I'm conveniently leaving out my own role in this tale of family bonding, but in truth, any one of us could get a citation for air pollution on one of these trips.

This kind of intimacy can be a challenge for couples to navigate, especially early on in a relationship, but children are already accustomed to having their parents inordinately involved in their bodily functions—we taught them how to *use* the bathroom, often by bribing them with candy—so they tend to be less self-conscious about these things. There is no slinking away, no feelings of shame. Dylan will grab the toilet bag and announce to the world, "I'm off to dig a hole!" as if he still expects to be rewarded with M&Ms upon his return.

While the hole-digging problems are universal, women have the added challenge of learning how to pee without soiling their clothes. It's tougher than men might imagine, given the unpredictable spray patterns we women have to contend with. Rowan had been struggling with this during our first few outings, so in an effort to be helpful, Chad bought her a "female urination device" to use on the trail. If he loves anything more than backpacking, it's shopping for backpacking equipment. Unfortunately, he didn't consult me before making this purchase. As soon as he opened it, I knew it wouldn't work.

I had expected the Pibella to be about the size of a kitchen funnel, maybe a respirator mask. A large catchment area is key. But the opening was roughly the size of a quarter, and it drained into an even narrower tube. Imagine trying to spray a garden hose through a drinking straw. Scratch that—imagine putting your thumb over the end of a garden hose and *then* trying to spray it through a drinking straw. That's how I imagined this working.

Chad saw my skepticism but persisted in his efforts to sell me on the device.

"You girls can pee standing up," he said cheerfully, as if this were news I'd been waiting my entire life to hear. It was true though—you *could* stand up and use the funnel. And you'd soak through your pants just the same as if you'd decided to let loose mid-stride.

In the end, I had to physically demonstrate for my daughter how to pee off trail. This was not the kind of bonding experience I had envisioned having with her when she was born, but it brought us closer nevertheless.

If nothing else, backpacking often reminds us that we need each other. I need my family to overlook my solo morning walks and to reassure me that every rustling in the bushes is not a cougar poised to attack us. The kids need us to provide them with the space to challenge themselves while feeling secure in the knowledge that we will be there to pick them up when they fall. It seems to me that all of these things could easily be accomplished within the city limits as well, but this is the life we've chosen for ourselves. It's a good one, despite my griping.

Whenever we reach the summit that we're tackling on each trip, I am momentarily relieved of both the physical and psychological burdens I felt on the trek up, and I understand why we put ourselves through such misery to get there. Being on high ground has its benefits.

As we survey the landscape below, sweaty and exhausted from our journey, I'll put my arms around the kids and remember holding them when they were born, when the experience was nearly identical: I was spent and exhilarated and had pooped in full view of other people just the same. I hope they are able to see the struggles I contend with to be able to stand there with them, that they feel inspired to do the things that scare them. I hope they feel pride in their own accomplishments and that they never feel shame to have a body that functions exactly as it was intended to. And, above all else, I hope to God that they keep their father from ever eating the gumbo.

27

Grin and Bear It

Over breakfast this morning, Dylan and I were reviewing how to respond to wild animal encounters in the backcountry, thanks to a panic-inducing article about wilderness safety that Google saw fit to start my day with.

"Should you find yourself being attacked by a grizzly bear," I reminded him, disregarding the fact that we don't have grizzlies in our neck of the woods, "lie flat on your stomach with your legs spread wide so that it can't flip you over and eviscerate you."

Dylan made a face but nodded in understanding, then resumed eating his oatmeal without a care. I, on the other hand, was instantly and deeply absorbed in this vision of being mauled to death by a bear. The scenario played out so vividly in my mind that my heart began racing, and my palms started to sweat.

"I wonder how long you remain conscious when an animal starts to eat you," I said, to no one in particular.

Dylan continued eating but managed a simple "That's. .

.horrifying" between bites. Had I just paused for a moment to consider how much this conversation would eventually cost me in therapy bills for my son, I might have ended here. But I made no such mental calculations and instead doubled down on this little horror show I was concocting.

"I should carry a vial of cyanide around my neck or something so that I can just die quickly if I'm being eaten." In my head, I was wondering if I should mention that I wasn't sure if cyanide would kill me any faster than having my guts ripped out, because it felt important to get the science right. Kids absorb so much.

The cyanide line was the one that finally got Dylan to stop eating. I couldn't decipher the look on his face—it was an odd amalgam of concern, fascination, and disgust—and I suddenly wished I hadn't given him this insight into my private thoughts.

"If you could just *faint*," he said, suggesting this was something I ought to be able to do on command, "then being eviscerated wouldn't be too bad." He was satisfied enough with this commentary to resume eating, as relaxed as if he had just returned from a stint in an ashram. Meanwhile, the conversation had provoked an anxiety attack so severe I briefly thought I might faint at the breakfast table, with nary a bear in sight.

It's so clear to me in watching my children, who seem to suffer none of the racing or intrusive thoughts or the physical manifestations of anxiety I've dealt with all of my life, that they have been spared whatever genetic quirk I was gifted in order to become the neurotic mess I am today. Whenever my anxiety threatens to overwhelm me—which it seems to regularly these days—I can at least take some comfort in knowing the kids won their father's Norwegian stoicism in their genetic lottery.

But small comforts just never add up to much whenever you're dealing with a clinically significant medical problem. I finally had to face this fact recently when I realized all of the techniques I have learned through the years to manage my anxiety were no longer working for me. My body was responding to various triggers before my mind even had a chance to register that something worth worrying about was happening. It's impossible to stop and reframe your thinking when your reptile brain has gotten your body to believe a bear is always standing by, licking its chops.

Still, I couldn't stand the thought of being medicated as a matter of routine, and I continued to resist. I visited my general practitioner for a physical just to see if something in my bloodwork might indicate that I was suffering from something other than a mental problem. It wasn't the stigma of mental illness that led to this thinking—I've always been forthright about my struggles with anxiety and depression—I just don't think the medical establishment has a firm grasp on how psychotropic drugs even work. Plus, I told the doctor I had tried several kinds of medication in the past, but they caused side effects that I just couldn't tolerate. I had intended to leave the "side effects" comment vague, but the doctor pressed me on this.

"What kind of side effects?" he asked, typing away on his computer.

I sighed and squirmed in my seat.

"Sexual ones." I hoped this would be enough for charting purposes, but apparently it was not.

"And what kind of sexual side effects did you experience?"

Because this was my first visit with this particular provider and because he was a man of about my age who happens to live in my neighborhood and is only one degree removed from my social circle, I didn't really want to tell him the problem. But he was leaving me no choice.

I had to say, out loud, that these medications left me unable to achieve an orgasm. The word seemed to echo in the room *Orgasm! Orgasm! Orgasm!* bouncing off the T-Rex stickers that were plastered on the walls, making my declaration all the more uncomfortable, even if it would seem that the T-Rex, with its uselessly short arms for any kind of self-pleasure, could at least feel my pain. But it had to be said. I just couldn't have one while medicated—not solo, not with a partner, not in a group—nothing. As someone who has always been, shall we say, easy to please, I found this too frustrating to take.

And what did that say about me, I wondered? I felt like this admission was tantamount to sticking my head out of the window and yelling to the world I LOVE ORGASMS, because I was, in essence, saying I'd rather live life in a constant state of mild panic than live without them. I was mortified to be having this conversation. The doctor, however, was unfazed and simply told me this was fairly typical of the drugs that were most effective for anxiety and moved on.

It's been nearly twenty years since I last tried medication, so I was disappointed to learn that no progress has been made in that time that would allow an anxious person to climax without being simultaneously preoccupied with nuclear holocaust. But I suppose there have been more pressing issues to attend to—such as nuclear holocaust.

My bloodwork came back normal, so I had to face the simple fact that my brain was to blame for my struggles, and if I wanted to feel better, I was going to have to try the drugs again. But I had one final Hail Mary pass to make before I relented: the all-natural hippie cure-all known as CBD.

CBD is all the rage these days, touted as a remedy for everything from arthritis to depression. It's the bland cousin of THC, which is the compound in marijuana that causes its characteristic high, but because CBD is derived from hemp, research on its health benefits has, until recent years, been strictly regulated by the federal government. The few studies that have been conducted suggest it could be useful in the treatment of anxiety disorders, so I pinned all of my hopes for a calm mind and plentiful orgasms on this substance.

Here in Washington State, where even recreational marijuana is legal, CBD shops are nearly as ubiquitous as Starbucks, so it wasn't difficult to find a supplier. I stopped into a shop one afternoon and explained to the proprietor that my goal was to reduce my general level of anxiety, and I asked if he had any personal experience with his products.

"Oh yeah. This works great for anxiety," he said, pointing to a bottle of bright orange gummies. "I take these every day and feel super chill."

It's probably worth noting this man smelled like he'd just been in a street fight with Pepé Le Pew, so I doubted it was the CBD that was responsible for his blissed-out state. Nevertheless, I was desperate, so I took the one that also contained ginger and turmeric extract so that I could at least get some anti-inflammatory benefits if the CBD didn't do anything.

When I returned home and resolved to try my first gummy, I immediately hit a snag: though there had been a plastic wrapping around the bottle cap, there was no inner foil lining over the bottle's opening. I tried to think of any other pill or vitamin that did not have a protective layer over the mouth of the container, but I could not. Because I am old enough to remember the tainted Tylenol incident of the early 1980s, I immediately believed I was in possession of a bottle of poison, and, naturally, I panicked.

I tried sniffing the gummies, but since I had no idea what they should have smelled like, this was of no use. I looked up all of the information I could find about this particular brand of CBD online, but no one had ever posted anything about the packaging, nor were there any images available for me to check my bottle against. I tried using the company's live chat to ask if this was a packaging problem or if the pills were supposed to come without an inner seal, but the question must have been ridiculous enough that it didn't warrant an answer. When I explained my concerns to my husband, he delicately suggested my reaction might be evidence that I needed the help of real medicine.

Fair enough. I knew I was being slightly irrational. But I also knew people had died from the cyanide-laced Tylenol, so I still thought it best to err on the side of caution. The next day, I stopped into the CBD shop again and asked the owner if the packaging came without that second seal.

"Oh yeah, that's totally normal," he said. "These hippie companies don't want to use any excess packaging if they can help it."

I could feel myself relax.

"Oh good," I said. "You must think I'm a little nuts, huh?"

He laughed. "Nah," he said, flopping onto the couch behind his cash register, the embodiment of chill, "We all have our little things, right?"

Little things, major neuroses—why quibble over semantics?

~

I took my first pill the next afternoon and went outside to do some weeding. I'm not sure how long I was working before I suddenly stopped and thought *I feel very calm.* Though CBD does not produce a high like THC and is generally not felt by its users unless they have a strong sedative response to it, I so rarely feel relaxed that this sensation registered as something foreign. I took a few deep breaths, chalked the feeling up to the placebo effect, and returned to my weeding.

The next morning, I took another pill before sitting down to do the crossword. It was coffee hour for me, so I didn't expect the CBD to be able to counteract the effects of all the caffeine I put in my system, but again, maybe a half hour or so after taking it, I looked up from my puzzle and realized this same calm feeling had overtaken me. It was some combination of the lightness I feel after meeting a deadline and the muscular looseness I feel after a hot bath. I recognized this feeling from the previous afternoon, and I suddenly understood how profoundly anxiety had been affecting my body. I broke down sobbing and continued to sob off and on for an hour until my husband woke up, and I sobbed in his arms for ten minutes more. Finally, after so many years, I felt *relief*.

As my CBD experiment wore on, I began making mental notes about situations that would normally have sent a jolt of panic through my body but now seemed subdued. Sirens had been anxiety provoking for the last several months, as had the sounds of C-17s flying overhead on approach to McChord. Now, they were provoking little more than mild annoyance.

Then, while driving on the highway, which is typically a high-stress situation for me, I took note of a speeding car that was about to pass by. In the recent past, the sound of the approaching car alone would have started my heart racing. In this instance, the sound merely alerted me to the car's approach. I marveled at this as I told my husband.

"I still can't believe I didn't react to that in my *body*." I shook my head as I drove.

"I'm so sorry you've been living this way," he said, reaching over to touch my knee.

"Don't distract the driver," I teased, swatting him away.

~

It's clear to me now, as either the CBD or the placebo effect has succeeded in muting my panic, that I had been living with my fight-or-flight response almost constantly activated, which is why my cognitive behavioral therapy techniques were no longer working for me. The brain struggles with rational thought when it enters this primal survival mode, and everything, even seemingly insignificant things, can trigger panic or, at times, rage. I can only imagine my depressive episodes over the last several years have been my body's desperate attempt to interrupt this stress response—a primitive system, perhaps, but one that likely kept me from dying of a heart attack.

Will this feeling last? It's impossible to know. At the very least it's been instructive for me to experience feeling calm again so that I might someday be able to access this state without the help of a magic pill. Now that I am less agitated overall, when I do still feel the slight shock of panic, I am better equipped to face it with the tools I've acquired in therapy. I am embracing every moment I have feeling this way. Mindfulness is far easier when your mind is not a whirling tornado of catastrophe.

~

Later this summer, I have made plans to hike to the crater rim of Mount Saint Helens with my family, a trip that will take us from the disquietingly named town of Cougar, through bear country, up to the mouth of an active volcano.

"If I had planned this trip, you would have been *pissed*," Chad joked. I could only nod in agreement. It's the kind of trip I would have white-knuckled my way through in the past, but one I'm actually looking forward to now as a way to prove my commitment to overcoming anxiety. If I were the dramatic sort, I might take my CBD to the top of the mountain just to hurl it into the steaming crater, as if somewhere in the journey I had claimed victory over my demons. But without it, I fear I might not be able to get back down—not yet, anyway. Baby steps. In this moment, just *wanting* to look into that abyss, to know I can even think of standing there, is all the victory I need.

28

Animal Natures

My cousin stopped by while on a cross-country drive from North Carolina a while back, and as we sipped iced tea on my porch, she told me that when she was a child, she used to enjoy watching my father put chickens to sleep. At first I thought she was using this term "put to sleep" euphemistically —we did kill and eat our chickens after all—but she assured me that he was actually just knocking them unconscious for a bit. She demonstrated how he'd cradle the bird like a baby, tuck its head in under the wing, then rock it to sleep.

"Like so," she said, jerking her arms back and forth. "It'd pass right out."

"I think you mean he gave it a concussion," I said.

She shrugged her shoulders. "Probably. But it's not like there's much going on inside a chicken's head."

I could hardly protest my father's treatment of the chickens. I had, myself, once drown almost an entire batch of peeps when I decided to give them a bath that involved simply submerging them in a bucket of water and holding them there.

I was very young at the time, too young to know that what I was doing would kill them, but probably old enough to know that I should have felt bad as I watched my parents desperately try to revive them with a hair dryer. But I did not.

I had a complex relationship with animals as a child. We ate most of the livestock that we raised on our hobby farm, but I still treated them like pets, even though I routinely watched my father dress their carcasses and was held rapt by the anatomy lessons he would give me as he worked.

"Oh look! Laverne and Shirley still had poop in their intestines!" I'd say, examining the entrails of the rabbits I had been cuddling mere hours before. I couldn't tell you why my father was bothering to kill the rabbits in the first place, since we had animals of more substance to stock our freezer with. Still, I thought nothing of it, as if it were a perfectly normal way to spend an afternoon, squeezing poop pellets through my dead rabbit's digestive tract until they fell into the grass at my feet.

I didn't mind the barnyard dissections, but I couldn't bring myself to watch any of the animals go to slaughter save for the chickens. I actually enjoyed watching them get the ax. It wasn't because they would terrorize me with their frantic pecking whenever I'd collect eggs from the coop—I wasn't vindictive—it was just fun to watch their headless bodies take off running across the yard. Chicken culling was entertainment, pure and simple, and I realize now that by not just participating but *delighting* in it, I no longer have the moral authority to judge anyone for watching the *Real Housewives of Orange County*.

I imagine most people who have lived on a farm or hunted

for their food have trouble with our modern tendency to assign human traits to animals and to pamper them as if they were children. To them, animals have utility. They put money in the bank and food on the table. To lavish time and money on them without hope of financial return is either an inexcusable extravagance or evidence of simple foolishness. Probably both.

My father would never have believed that city folk keep hens after their laying years have passed, just feeding them as if they were pets instead of the used-up freeloaders that they really are. We had enough of those types in the family already to willingly add more to the mix.

I often wonder what my father would think of the way my family treats our dog—how any family with some disposable cash and time on their hands treats a dog for that matter. While we don't dress ours in designer clothes or send her to posh dog resorts when we go on vacation, we are perhaps a bit overly attentive to her needs, especially in the diet department.

"You feed it *what?*" I can imagine my father saying before sampling the dog's duck and oatmeal kibble (he was never too particular about cuisine). I'll admit the dog eats better than I did as a kid, when my idea of a treat was a tin of Vienna sausages eaten cold. But she's a city dog who has never known a day of work in her life and as a result has developed a taste for the finer things.

The farm dogs were not so lucky. Not only were my child-hood dogs decidedly not pampered, they were, to some extent, expendable. Bad behavior wasn't tolerated or addressed with a dog trainer. Farm dogs were just. . .dealt with. When my two labs Corky and Scruffy began running off to the neighbor's farm to get into his chicken coop, for example, my father simply took them out to the woods and shot them. Since the dogs tended to roam anyway, he told me that they ran off and never came back. This explanation must have satisfied me.

Months later, while playing at the edge of the woods along the cow pasture, I came across two perfect animal skulls—unthinkable treasures for a kid—and raced back to the house to show them to my mother. I don't remember the look on her face as I held up the remains of the "runaway" dogs, but it probably said something like, "There's not enough therapy in the world to fix this."

My mother obviously didn't let me keep the skulls, nor did she tell me about their origins, but before she could dispose of them, I pulled the teeth out of the jaw bones and stashed them in a box under my bed. I can't even begin to imagine where this impulse came from. This is exactly the sort of story people recount about serial killers.

"She seemed normal enough. But I heard she pried the teeth out of her dead dogs' jaws and slept with them under her pillow," someone would say years later, when I was finally apprehended by law enforcement for some unspeakable crime. "It's always the quiet ones."

I didn't find out until much later that the skulls belonged to my pets. I find the fact that I kept the teeth darkly hilarious, but the story never seems to elicit laughter whenever I tell it at parties, only a pensive assessment of me as a person. I can almost see people's thoughts as they process what I've told them. *Ah,* their faces seem to say. Now *I understand you.*

~

If an animal could ever be said to have understood me, it would have been my dog Chino. I adopted him while I was in the clutches of grief over my father's suicide, at a time when I was in no frame of mind to do such a thing. *I couldn't save my father, but I can at least save a dog,* I remember thinking when I got him. I was at least partially aware of the flaws in this logic, but I was undeterred. My husband hadn't been keen on the idea at the time, so I gave him two options: "I'm getting a dog or a lover," I'd said. Within months we both realized I had chosen poorly.

Chino had been a troubled dog from the beginning. He was anxious and territorial, always miserably on edge—basically the dog version of me. This kinship solidified our bond and ours alone. While I had known him to be a loving companion, he was protective of me and suspicious to the point of aggression. Everyone else in my house saw him as a ticking time bomb.

I had tried everything under the sun to rehabilitate this animal: medication, hours of daily exercise, a special diet. I even spent an outrageous amount of money on a trainer who specialized in training dogs for both law enforcement and personal protection to see if she could pinpoint the root of his aggression and offer us some hope. I had fallen into that trap of inexcusable extravagance or utter foolishness. My father wouldn't have hesitated to call my choices foolish.

Chino had been doing well with his training, but after an unprovoked attack on my daughter, even the trainer had to level with me, offering the same advice I'm sure my father would have given me months and months earlier: *Sometimes putting an animal down is the humane thing to do.*

It's difficult not to draw parallels between the dog's mental illness and my father's, to anthropomorphize the animal to such an extent that it became a surrogate for my father, a being onto whom I could project all of my unspent love and care and naïve hope for recovery and redemption. But maybe the dog and I had formed some kind of understanding all the while. Maybe he knew I was the one who could truly know the depths of his suffering.

When I came to terms with the fact that I was fighting a losing battle with Chino, I remember wishing I could have called my father for reassurance. He'd have joked with me to put me at ease. He'd have reminded me that dogs will eat their owners who die alone at home. He'd have said that loyalty is just a construct. But that I already knew.

It's been years at this point, but I still sometimes wish I could view my father's death—even the dog's death—the way I used to view the deaths of the animals on the farm: an inevitable conclusion, unremarkable and routine. A release from a world that was never particularly kind. In the end, it was that concept of release—of relief—that allowed me to say goodbye.

When I finally put the dog down eighteen months after I adopted him, I did so with resignation and with what I believed—beyond reason—was both his and my father's other-worldly approval. Maybe it was the right and necessary thing. Maybe I failed them both. Either way, I learned that the only one I could ever hope to save in this life was myself.

Epilogue

And you, Dear Reader—

If you are struggling to save yourself from self-destructive thoughts, please contact the good people at the National Suicide Prevention Lifeline: 1-800-273-8255.

Don't give up hope. You are loved beyond measure.

And seriously, your dog will eat you.

29

Notes & Asides

Consider these notes callbacks, codas, post-credit scenes—whatever you like. They may be read alone or in conversation with the original piece.

Make, Model, and Class

". . .a high I'd only previously felt from my codeine-laced cough syrup."

Medical professionals of the 1970s and early 1980s seemed hell-bent on getting children stoned. There was codeine in our garden variety over-the-counter cough syrup, and my husband and I could both swear that we each had a vial of liquid cocaine in our medicine cabinets, readily accessible to anyone who might suffer from a fatal bout of curiosity. You know, like a child.

Drugging children was so pervasive that my childhood dentist Dr. Livengood (yes, Livengood) gassed me with nitrous at every single appointment. I must have been given such high doses that I've been left with only hazy impressions of my visits with him. The only real memory I have of the dentist is of a cheery female voice saying "Time to put on the space mask!" as the device closed in on my face. God only knows what was happening to me while I was out. I could have been a practice patient for every dental student in Western Pennsylvania for all I know. But at least I was compliant.

"Poor kids rarely realize they're poor. . ."

It's worth noting here that we were poor at this time because my father had left and largely failed to pay child support. My mother worked while she went back to school to become an x-ray technician, clawing her way out of poverty on her own. She succeeded in the face of grim odds, and I admire her for it.

". . .Catholic schools didn't cater to the children from the monied families necessarily. . ."

In my children's old private school, it was perfectly clear who had the money. There's a fair amount of one-upmanship that happens in any community, I realize, but private-school parents can truly take it to the next level. Take Flat Stanley for example. For those of you who don't have children, allow me to explain. Flat Stanley is a children's book character who is accidentally flattened by a falling bulletin board in his sleep, and rather than despair over his predicament, he takes advantage of his new slender profile to travel the world through the postal service. Elementary school children send their own paper Stanleys to friends and relatives all over the world, and he reports back to the class with tales of his adventures. Naturally, this provides a perfect opportunity for certain parents to show off their connections. The reports that came in from my children's classmates went something like this:

"My Flat Stanley visited the governor," one child reported.

"My Flat Stanley visited the President," said another.

"MY Flat Stanley visited the SPACE STATION!" another would counter, and so on, ad infinitum.

Meanwhile, our Flat Stanley went four-wheeling to a meat raffle in Minnesota.

It was a fantasy meritocracy I had imagined all those years ago after all.

Screen Times

". . .I loved spending time with [television characters] more than their real-life human equivalents."

The one notable exception to this was Fred Flintstone, who inspired a mortal terror that persists to this day. The episode that scarred me was a spoof of a James Bond movie. It featured a scheming villain named Dr. Sinister and his seductive assistant Madame Yes, who lured Fred and Barney into the doctor's lair inside of a remote island volcano. Once there, Dr. Sinister threatened to throw them into something he called simply "the pit." I vaguely recall some background character yelling out "Not the pit!" to underscore the horror of this fate, at which point Dr. Sinister threw a boulder into the abyss and told Fred and Barney to listen.

"I don't hear anything," Fred said, his voice in a quiver.

"That's because it's bottomless," Dr. Sinister replied.

"You mean we just keep falling?"

"That's right," Dr. Sinister said. "Forever and Ever and EVER!"

He let out an evil cackle, prompting me, at my tender young age, to completely crack. I came undone at the thought of Fred falling *forever* in that darkness. It's a feeling I now get from science fiction movies when astronauts come untethered and float off into the vacuum of space, but in that moment, this idea of the void was one I had not yet encountered.

There was too much for me to unpack. First, I had to wrestle with the notion of something being endless. That was difficult enough. I had already been struggling to understand the concept of eternity when I thought about spending that amount of time burning in a lake of fire in the afterlife. But I also had to grapple with the question of Fred's mortality. He eventually would have to die, perhaps after years and years of falling, at which point his lifeless body would continue to fall forever, the pit itself his only destination. I shudder from the memory alone.

Unlocking Your Unlimited Potential

I unearthed the unsavory bits of Barrie Konicov's life on his Wikipedia page.

I have yet to master astral projection.

All Signs Point to Death

"I recite the same few lines of poetry during takeoff every time I fly in order to keep the plane aloft."

Then I would ease my anxiety with alcohol. On one trip that I took while my husband was at the controls, the head flight attendant had seemingly made it her mission in life to get me absolutely wasted, I can only assume to help me relax. At one point, after serving me several generous glasses of wine, she invited me up to the first-class area to give me a glass of champagne and strawberries as she spritzed my face with rose water.

We were standing in the galley area behind the flight deck, and I was probably making a big production of the face spritzing, as one of the first-class passengers had stopped reading his newspaper to watch the scene unfold. I'll never forget the look on his face as he peered up at us over his bifocals, a cross between anticipation and disbelief, an unspoken "My God this *does* happen in real life!" kind of look.

So, it isn't really just the poetry that calms me whenever I fly. The champagne and strawberries and faintly homoerotic encounters with flight attendants help some, too.

A Valentine for My ENT

". . .awkwardly crooning 'I love you, platonically love youuuuu' to the tune of Olivia Newton John's 'I Honestly Love You'."

I am constantly making up words to old songs to narrate my daily life. But sometimes I simply sing old tunes that fit the task at hand. Every time I pull fresh loaves of bread from the oven, for example, I sing "Baby Imma Want You," and no one in my family appreciates how hilarious this is. If you get this joke, let's be friends.

The AI in Anxiety

My mother kept a small black-and-white television set on the kitchen counter in my childhood home. It had a dial with about twelve channels that we could use to tune into the public networks, along with a UHF tuner that we never bothered with, since we could never pick up any broadcasts over those channels.

One night at dinner, I was fiddling with the UHF dial when I discovered that I could pick up conversations on some of the frequencies—truckers on their CB radios, for example, or neighbors chatting about the weather on their wireless telephones nearby. This immediately became our nightly source of entertainment. Occasionally there was the hint of something scandalous going on, but mostly the talk was mundane. While some families were tuning into the evening news as a backdrop to their dinner, we were spying on our neighbors. It seems so quaint now, this form of spying. Who could have predicted there would come a day when people would offer up all of the information I was listening to in secret—and then some.

It was quite possibly the most fun I've ever had with my family.

Life is but a Dream

Descartes, Rene. *Meditations on First Philosophy.* 1641.
Try making sense of the Static Theory of Time here:
https://plato.stanford.edu/entries/time/#DynaStatTheo.

Finding Your Voice

Flight 412 from Seattle to Pittsburgh was delayed the morning I set off for my research trip, and as I waited, I glanced at my watch only to find that the battery had died earlier in the night—at 4:12 to be exact. I made a mental note to buy a lottery ticket with the numbers. When the plane finally boarded, the pilot announced that our flying time would be four hours and twelve minutes, with an ETA of just after 4:00 pm. At that point I was completely convinced that we were going to crash and die upon landing, thus making my stopped watch an omen. We survived, but we did arrive at the gate at exactly 4:12 pm. If you also suffer from anxiety, you understand what a nightmare such coincidences are.

An Essay Concerning Avian Understanding

I have always been fond of watching birds. As a child, I was particularly taken with the cardinals that would frequent my grandfather's yard, and my family dubbed the whole of them "Joanna's redbird," as if they were mine alone to protect and attend to, possession the natural consequence of my affection. No one thought to tell me we can never really hold what we love.

To me, cardinals will always be the symbol of simple times and easy joy. I still feel a small thrill whenever I am fortunate enough to see one. They were a comfort to me during a few strange and lonely years in Delaware, where they would flock to my trees—sometimes nine at a time—reminding me that there is always beauty to be found, even in the starkest of winters.

The cardinals are notably absent from my life now. Occasionally, a yellow warbler or scrub jay will brighten my yard, but over time, I have come to accept my view of the more muted and unassuming birds of the Pacific Northwest.

But I will never stop missing my redbird.

One winter, while in Baltimore visiting my grandfather, I joined him at his kitchen window to watch the birds peck at his feeders. I asked him if he saw cardinals very often, like he used to at his house in Pennsylvania. He shook his head. No, the blue jays were too territorial and kept them at bay. Just then, in a scene I would not have written into a story for fear of it being wholly unbelievable, a streak of crimson flew past us and settled into a nearby tree. I could barely stammer out "Look—" as I grabbed my grandfather's shoulder and pointed.

He didn't say a word. He didn't need to. Memories resurfaced with such force that we were time travelers in that moment, all the years gone, leaving us standing there in that Pennsylvania house as we once were or perhaps always will be. My uncle Craig and my father had not yet killed themselves; my grandmother, unaware yet that she, too, was dying, happily baked a cream cake for Christmas. Everyone was together. The first snow was pristine. Blue jays were of no concern to us yet, and the melt, with its mud and detritus, would come later. But as we looked out into the yard that day, everyone had gathered together with us, delivered through time to our memories, and delighted in the miracle of a cardinal in winter.

~

Information about Old Tom came from the *Scientific American* article below.

Crew, Bec. "The Legend of Old Tom and the Gruesome 'Law of the Tongue.'" *Scientific American*. June 4, 2014. https://blogs.scientificamerican.com/running-ponies/the-legend-of-old-tom-and-the-gruesome-law-of-the-tongue/

Captain Cook's Revenge

"I generally don't mind being on the water but I'm not fond of being in the water. . ."

Actually, I only like being near certain types of water. I've never been fond of ocean beaches. Apart from enjoying the sight of my children at play, the discomfort of the setting is nearly unbearable. The very moment I set foot on a beach, I have sand in my swim suit. I'm not sure of the physics behind this—maybe it's some kind of quantum phenomenon—but it is the one thing I absolutely know to be true in life: I will always leave the beach with enough sand in my bottom to prepare me for a career as a drug mule. If you like the beach, we can't be friends.

The Doctor Will See You Now

Strep throat seemed to be as routine as the common cold when my husband and I were young, which genuinely perplexes us both now, since neither of our children has ever had a case of it. When I was about three or four years old, seeing my doctor for what would become an annual shot of penicillin, he unceremoniously rolled me over, yanked down my pants and pierced me right in the rear without so much as a warning. As soon as I could wriggle free from him, I ran outside screaming, then pulled my own pants down, craning my neck to see if the needle had left a hole in my cheek. This episode seems to have set the tone for every subsequent medical visit of my life. I have yet to forgive him for this.

Don't Burst My Bubble

Giant bubble recipe:

1 gal water

5 c dish soap

1/2 c glycerin

Mix gently without creating bubbles in the solution. Let rest for 24 hours. Have fun!

A Christmas Miracle

On occasion, my husband will also have an awkward encounter that leaves me genuinely feeling less alone in the world. Take this for example: One morning, mid-pandemic, Chad had an ill-timed coughing fit while in Starbucks. A slight tickle in his throat suddenly morphed into a full-throated choke the minute he set foot in the store, and the sensation of coughing through a mask must have been mildly panic inducing, because in that moment he lacked the where-withal to simply excuse himself from the store to finish hacking up his lungs outside. The barista was not amused.

"I think she would have judged me less if I had been

robbing the place," he said when he returned to the car, red faced and wheezing.

His cough had not subsided. At one point he coughed so deeply that it actually activated *my* gag reflex, which prompted him to gag in response. I laughed so hard at this image of us tandem gagging in our car while parked in the Starbucks parking lot that I induced a tearful coughing fit of my own. The motorcyclist parked next to us could only look on in horror as two people were apparently dying of COVID before his very eyes.

We eventually pulled ourselves together and continued on with our day. Meanwhile, Starbucks took away all of our stars and banned us from its stores for life.

Cowboy Songs

Storm clouds were gathering in the distance as we crossed the border into Wyoming during an epic two-week family road trip through Yellowstone and the Tetons a few summers ago. The sight of the clouds reminded me of something I had read in Gretel Ehrlich's memoir *Match to the Heart*:

"Wyoming has the highest number of lightning strikes per capita," I announced to everyone in the car. This bit of trivia was met not with thoughtful silence but with an outright stone-cold refusal to acknowledge what I said. Chad and the kids have long stopped wondering why I have such information always at the ready, but you haven't, so now you have learned a fun fact for the day. Be careful out there on the range during storm season.

On the Burdens of Sex

Brockell, Gillian. "The 10th president's last surviving grandson: A bridge to the nation's complicated past." *The Washington Post.* November 29, 2020.

Tan, Rebecca. "This 74-year-old woman just gave birth to twins." *The Washington Post.* September 6, 2019.

Shifting the Gaze

"I always wondered how men run with their particular anatomy in the first place. . ."

After watching the American male sprinters run in the 2020 Olympics, I no longer have to wonder about this. Their uniforms left absolutely nothing to the imagination, and watching the slow-motion replays of the races with my family was easily one of the most uncomfortable experiences of my life. Google this at your own risk.

On the Trail Again

Backpacking Chicken Gumbo
This is slightly less toxic than the pre-packaged backpacking meals, but you should still proceed with caution. We use a recipe from the Appalachian Trail website thetrek.co/appalachian-trail/

Ingredients:
1 cup instant brown rice
½ cup dehydrated chicken *
½ cup dehydrated okra

¼ cup dehydrated onions

¼ cup dehydrated bell peppers

¼ cup dehydrated corn

¼ cup tomato sauce (leather or powder)

½ tsp garlic

½ tsp basil

½ tsp pepper

½ tsp cayenne pepper

¼ tsp thyme

2 bouillon cubes

Directions

1. Combine all ingredients in a vacuum sealed bag.

2. On the trail, pour ingredients into a pot. Add 3 cups of water and let sit for 5 minutes.

3. Bring to a boil and cook for 2 minutes.

*We generally dehydrate canned chicken for backpacking meals.

Grin and Bear It

Since my father was fond of grand gestures, I decided it would be appropriate to bring him along on our Mount Saint Helens hike so that I could toss some of his ashes into the crater as part of the farewell tour I've slowly been taking him on for the last several years. As I packed up for the trip, taking care to double wrap the baggie containing his remains, I found myself singing my own lyrics to John Denver's "Leaving on a Jet Plane." It went something like this: "Oh my dad is packed/ he's ready to go/ be thrown into/ a volcano."

Perhaps you find this irreverent. My father would have

found it hilarious. And he would have been proud of me for facing my fears and making the trek, for trying to be better, to evolve our family line. I like to think he would have appreciated bearing witness to this particular journey.

We did make the summit on our climb. A raven that had been following us up the mountain had perched itself on a cairn that someone had erected at the crater's edge, and I took that as a sign that this was where my father wanted to be. It was an uncharacteristically windless, bluebird kind of day, Spirit Lake and Mount Tahoma prominent in the background. Silly as it may sound, it felt as though the mountain had been waiting for my father, maybe even for me.

As I scattered the ashes into the steaming crater, I thought of that biblical lake of fire that had terrified me as a child, and I laughed at the irony of throwing my father into a literal version of it for his final resting place. But I realized he had already been forged in fire in this life, made razor sharp but brittle, like the obsidian that forms along the edges of a lava flow, stone I'd like to believe his ashes might meld with during Saint Helens' next eruption.

"I hope you enjoy the view, Dad," I said as I watched the cloud of ash drift into the crater, reflecting on all the ways we both had been transformed.

Acknowledgements

"Captain Cook's Revenge" first appeared, in slightly different form, in the *Tacoma News Tribune*.

Pieces of "Oh Captain, My Captain" first appeared in my *Thrive Global* essay titled "The Gift of Presence."